Reducing the Cost of Dental Care

Publications in the Health Sciences

Publication of this book was assisted by a
McKnight Foundation grant to the
University of Minnesota Press's program
in the health sciences.

Reducing the Cost of Dental Care

Robert T. Kudrle and Lawrence Meskin

Editors

University of Minnesota Press □ Minneapolis

Contributors

Howard L. Bailit, D.M.D. Professor, Department of Behavioral Sciences and Community Health, University of Connecticut School of Dental Medicine, Farmington, CT

Jeffrey C. Bauer, Ph.D. Coordinator of Program and Policy Analysis, Office of the Chancellor, University of Colorado Health Sciences Center and Associate Professor, Department of Applied Dentistry, University of Colorado School of Dentistry, Denver, CO

David O. Born, Ph.D. Professor, Department of Health Ecology, School of Dentistry, University of Minnesota, Minneapolis, MN

Brian A. Burt, B.D.Sc., M.P.H., Ph.D. Program in Dental Public Health, School of Public Health, The University of Michigan, Ann Arbor, MI

Douglas A. Conrad, Ph.D. Associate Professor, Departments of Community Dentistry and Health Services, University of Washington, Seattle, WA

Robert T. Kudrle, Ph.D. Associate Professor, Hubert Humphrey Institute of Public Affairs, University of Minnesota, Minneapolis, MN

Marvin Marcus, D.D.S. Professor, School of Dentistry, University of California—Los Angeles, Los Angeles, CA

Lawrence Meskin, D.D.S., Ph.D. Dean, School of Dentistry, University of Colorado, Denver, CO

v

Peter Milgrom, D.D.S. Associate Professor and Chairman, Department of Community Dentistry, University of Washington, Seattle, WA

Sheldon Rovin, D.D.S., M.S. Professor and Chairman, Department of Dental Care Systems, School of Dental Medicine, and Associate Director, Leonard Davis Institute of Health Economics and National Health Care Management Center, University of Pennsylvania, Philadelphia, PA

Richard Scheffler, Ph.D. Associate Professor of Economics, Department of Economics, George Washington University, Washington, D.C.

Samuel J. Tobin. Health Economist, University of California—Los Angeles, Los Angeles, CA

Kenneth E. Warner, Ph.D. Department of Health Planning and Administration, School of Public Health, The University of Michigan, Ann Arbor, MI

Acknowledgments

In an era when national conferences usually have a single major underwriter, the symposium that generated this book stands out as a unique tribute to the energies and dedication of a number of individuals and organizations. Financial support for the conference, held September 25 and 26, 1980, at the University of Minnesota in Minneapolis, came from Delta Dental Plan of Minnesota, Onan A. Thompson, President; California Dental Service, Dr. Erik D. Olsen, President, and the University of Minnesota's Center for Health Services Research, Dr. John Kralewski, Director. The symposium was presented by the Office of Continuing Education (School of Dentistry) under the direction of Dr. H. D. Foglesong. We would also like to acknowledge the assistance of the staff of the University of Minnesota's Department of Health Ecology with special recognition to Therese Pash for her coordinating effort that resulted in the logistic success of the conference.

A special acknowledgment is made to Delta Dental Plan of Minnesota, and its President, Onan A. Thompson, for their additional contribution to assist in the publication of the conference proceedings.

Preface

Consistent yearly increases in the utilization of dental services in the United States have resulted in per capita expenditures of approximately $68.42 in 1980 with total expenditure of $15.9 billion. Despite such huge outlays, economists and policy analysts have paid little attention to the dental-care sector of the economy. Moreover, when economists and other social scientists have directed attention to dentistry, they often have generalized from studies of other parts of the health-care delivery system. Special features that characterize the economics of dental care often have been ignored. This book confronts this problem by examining in depth a key issue in the dental-care delivery system: the potential for cost reduction. To address this issue, arrangements for essays on six major topics relating to cost reduction were made with people who had a long-standing concern with dental costs and who had a substantial interest in the economics of dental care. This approach resulted in six chapters—each prepared jointly by a person whose principal attachment is to the profession of dentistry and by at least one health economist. In all chapters but one this collaboration resulted in joint authorship.

When the project was originally conceived, we were optimistic but not certain that the combined perspectives would result in a coherent and important contribution. Although we leave the final judgment to the reader, our view is that the effort has been a success. We hope the book will be useful to policy analysts in government, insurance, and universities as well as to practicing professionals.

ix

Contents

Introduction

Robert T. Kudrle and Lawrence Meskin

Dental disease is perhaps the most prevalent chronic malady of mankind, and it is rampant in industrial and developing countries alike.[1] But unlike the bewildering variety of diseases that the broader health care sector treats, dental disease is primarily limited to a few major types. Dental caries (decay) and periodontal (tissue surrounding the teeth) disease are the most common and can ultimately lead to tooth loss. While oral cancer does occur, its incidence is rare and most treatment takes place outside the dental care sector. Growth and development problems, the concern of the dental specialties of orthodontics (teeth straightening) and pedodontics (children's dentistry), represent the corrective rather than disease-treating aspects of dentistry. Corrective dentistry accounts for an increasingly large part of dental care expenditures.

Dental problems, while occasionally painful, are rarely fatal and may be relatively asymptomatic until they reach a serious stage. Hence, many persons delay dental care—sometimes until the problems are beyond repair. The typical lack of urgency lends intuitive appeal to the evidence that far more than poverty keeps people away from the dentist. Social background is a more powerful determinant of contact with the dental care system than with the health care system in general. Many persons are deterred by the time and distance involved in obtaining dental treatment. The fear of pain also keeps people out of the dental office. Other persons, under the misconception that they are not susceptible to dental disease, postpone visits until symptoms become unbearable.

People with higher-than-average incomes and levels of education use dental services more than others—even when the care is "free." All of these factors together make unsurprising an often-confirmed fact about dental insurance: while only half the U.S. population sees a dentist in any given year, the increase engendered by complete insurance coverage usually brings the utilization rate no higher than about 70 percent. Most dentists agree that good dental health requires dental visits at least once a year.

As in the broader health care system, there are concerns in dentistry about all three of the criteria typically used to evaluate health care delivery systems: cost, access, and quality, including the extent to which treatment actually increases the health status of the patient.[2] While this book will address primarily the cost issue, it is worthwhile to introduce some background regarding the other criteria.

ACCESS

At one level, geographic access to dental care looks very much like the case in medical care. The often-cited comparison in medicine is between New York and South Dakota, where the number of physicians per capita in the former state in the mid-seventies was 2.79 times the number in the latter. This is remarkably similar to the most extreme comparison for dentists in the same period: a 2.75 to 1 ratio between New York and Mississippi (the ratio for New York to South Dakota was 1.83 to 1.)[3] Yet these state figures conceal important geographic access differences. In 1973 there was a 378 percent difference in the per capita availability of physicians in cities with one million population or more compared to areas with no urban population, while the comparable figure for dentists was 158 percent.[4] This, of course, represents in part the enormous concentration of medical specialists in the urban areas of the country. This raises two more sharp contrasts between medicine and dentistry. Very little of the practice of dentistry takes place in hospitals, and about 85 percent of all dentists are general practitioners.

However, the geographical distribution of dentists is determined by more than the preferences of individual practitioners. Although dentists pass national written board examinations to demonstrate intellectual understanding of their subject just as doctors do, dentists also must pass very comprehensive clinical examinations given by state boards of dental examiners. There is little doubt that these examinations have been used to control entry into the profession in many states.[5]

Social-class access issues are more marked in dentistry than in medicine. In large part because of the unobtrusive nature of dental disease and the widely varying attitudes among social classes about the inevitability of tooth loss, education and income each play independent roles in determining who uses the dental care system. Racial differences also are substantial; blacks have much lower contact with the dental care system than do whites.

Some dental benefits are offered under Medicaid in nearly all states, yet the impact of Medicaid dental benefits on the dental health of poor people appears to be much more uncertain than Medicaid's impact on their overall health. Some states award benefits only to children, and no way has been devised to overcome client indifference to available services.[6]

QUALITY

International comparisons find the average quality of dental care in the United States to be very high. Yet dentists are subject to little peer observation in their work, and there is apparently great variation in the quality of services provided.[7] Furthermore, as in medicine, the patient is seldom able to make an accurate judgment about the quality of work performed. On the other hand, dentistry is better placed than is medicine to control quality if this were an overriding goal. Many problems and much treatment leave a record on hard tissue that is traceable by radiographs, a fact that has led to considerable monitoring by insurance companies of the necessity for treatment and sometimes its quality.[8]

Quality, construed as the reduction of dental disease, is a more difficult issue. There is little doubt that professional treatment contributes to improved dental health, yet the degree of improvement pales in statistical comparison with two other forms of intervention. Water fluoridation may reduce the incidence of dental caries by as much as two-thirds.[9] By contrast, the impact of most professionally administered "prevention" not involving fluoride on the incidence of caries is problematic. Professionally delivered prevention has a more established record in the area of periodontal disease, yet personal attention to oral hygiene is usually much more effective. A parallel with health care in general is apt: personal behavior often dominates professional intervention as a source of health. Yet, generally healthful behavior—a reduction in eating, smoking and drinking and the taking of exercise—is apparently deemed too high a price by most people for the increased probability of good health. The cost of preventive dental care is low, and regular careful brushing and flossing of the teeth results in a considerable reduction in expected periodontal disease.

But only a modest fraction of the U.S. population appears willing to pay the price. It is difficult to avoid the conclusion that many people just do not take dental health very seriously.

With this brief look at the access and quality situation in dentistry, we can approach the cost issue, with which this book will principally deal.

COST

Dentistry is a rapidly growing part of the U.S. economy. This was not always so. Between 1929 and 1950, the share of dentistry in total GNP dropped from 0.47 percent to 0.34 percent. By 1960, however, it was back up to 0.39 percent and by 1980 it had risen 76 percent above its 1950 share to 0.60 percent.[10] Moreover, during the seventies, dentistry maintained its share of rapidly rising health-care expenditures. Yet, there has been little of the public outcry about "uncontrollable" or "runaway" expenditures in dentistry that has accompanied the rather similar proportionate growth of total health care costs.

Two factors may explain the difference. One is absolute size: dental care is only about 6.4 percent of total U.S. health care expenditures. The other is the overwhelmingly private nature of dental care spending: while the state and national governments pay for about 40 percent of all health care expenditures, their relative share of dental expenditures is less than 4 percent.

Is the "cost" of dental care really a problem? What criteria should be used to answer the question? "Cost" has varying meanings. One is clearly the figure related to the various percentages reported above. This definition of cost is simply the quantity of services produced multiplied by their prices.

The burgeoning cost of health care in recent years has generated an almost universal call for "cost containment." This cry usually is a reaction to total public cost—a subset of total expenditures—that has dominated political discussions of health care and has given impetus for much public policy action. In dentistry the outcry has remained muted; public payment for dentistry amounts to only about 0.6 percent of total public health care outlays. This is not to say that public payments for dental care have been made with no attention to or concern about excessive cost. There have been enough verified cases of excessive or improper treatment under the Medicaid program to raise serious doubt in the minds of some public officials about the effectiveness of the present system of public payment for dental services.[11] And yet, because dentistry "isn't where the bucks are," public action has been slight. Most public officials think publicly financed dental care benefits can be curtailed with relatively mild client outcry. The sector is not regarded as one in which major efficiencies in service provision could be easily achieved. This stands in sharp contrast to much of the rest of the health care sector. Thus, government dental benefits are often seen principally as victims of the absence of cost control elsewhere in the publicly paid health-care system than as a major source of the problem.

Nearly everyone concerned with health care expenditures is concerned about both the volume and the price of services delivered, largely as separable issues. The volume of dental services has given most observers little problem. In contrast to the case of the broader health care sector, there is much concern on the part of those knowledgeable about dental health that overall public contact with the delivery system is vastly inadequate. Although there is some concern about excessive service and the provision of costly services where cheaper ones would do, it is difficult to identify large and systematic patterns of excess dental treatment comparable to excessive hospitalization and surgery.[12]

As with expenditures for dental services and their volume, little attention has been paid to dental-care prices. The physician-service index rose by 216 percent between 1960 and 1979; over the same period, the dental-service index increased by 162 percent. Some claim that this is a relatively good record; after all, over the same period the CPI rose by 145 percent.[13]

To the extent that the price indexes used adequately represent real price changes,[14] the unit price of dentistry does not appear to be performing badly. Yet, it is obvious that this is an incomplete picture. Anyone concerned with efficiency in the provision of dental care must be interested not only in changes in the price of services but with the price level itself. How much lower would dental care prices be if various technical, institutional and public policy innovations were in place?

This perspective suggests some additional crucial cost distinctions. (Table 1 presents some definitions helpful in the following discussion.) At the unit level, "cost" can refer to the price paid for the service, or to some measure of the unit costs experienced by the dental practice, or to the economist's definition of unit cost: real resource cost. Prices can be high because the real resource cost is high, or because the dentist faces artificially high prices for the inputs he buys, or because of the dentist's profits (taken either as money or as leisure). From

Table 1. Dental Cost Definitions

Term	Definition
Total Expenditure	Prices paid times quantity of dental services delivered over the entire economy.
Total Public Expenditure	Prices paid times quantity of dental services paid with public funds.
Unit Price	Amount paid for a unit of service.
Full Price	Unit price plus value of time involved in obtaining service.
Unit Cost	Amount of cost per unit experienced by dentistry.
Total Cost	Total cost experienced by dentistry.
Unit Opportunity Cost	Value of resources used in the production of a unit of service estimated as forgone economic value.
Total Opportunity Cost	The estimated value of all resources used in dentistry estimated as forgone value.

the purchaser's viewpoint, moreover, money price does not exhaust "cost." There is at least one other component: the value of the time involved in obtaining the service. The money price and the time price together are often called the "full price."

An example can help clarify some distinctions. Suppose dental hygienists use a labor organization to raise the fee for their services above the level necessary to train and hold people in their branch of the field. The difference between the new wage and the old one represents a "transfer payment" from patients and dentists to the auxiliaries involved but does not mean that more of society's resources are being used to produce dental services: it is simply a transfer of purchasing power.

The economist's use of the term "cost" refers to the value of resources used in the production of a good or service valued at the "opportunity cost" of those resources: the dollar value of opportunities forgone in the rest of the economy to produce the dental service. To continue our example: if the cost of hygienists' services increases—not because of any monopoly elements in the labor market but because of the alternative uses of the time of persons involved increase in value—this is a "real" increase in cost.

Only completely competitive conditions can ensure that price is equal to real resource cost for a unit of a firm's production, and this raises perhaps the most relevant distinction of all between price and real resource cost: that between the costs experienced by the dentist, including a competitive return on his labor and education, and the prices he charges. While the American system usually relies on market forces to keep prices and costs in line, we cannot simply assume that those forces are always operating to maximum effect. Economists investigating dentistry have adduced evidence to support the view that dentistry has earned excess profits for many years, meaning simply that average net incomes of dentists could be substantially lowered without an important effect on the willingness of persons to become or remain dentists.[15] These extra profits have been explained by the lack of competition among dentists. This situation has been made possible largely by professionally sponsored restrictions on advertising and by limitations on the number of persons trained as dentists. Whether the new legality of dental advertising (see discussion below) and the rapidly increasing dentist-population ratio will diminish or eliminate estimated "excess" profits in dentistry remains to be seen. The concomitant reduction in prices (both money and "full") would be a very real cost reduction from the standpoint of the consumer.

By extension, total costs either experienced by dental firms or estimated as opportunity costs are two additional applications of the term "cost" to dentistry.

It is quite likely that a decrease in dental prices for uninsured persons would lead to an increase in total expenditure by them, which appears to mean that one kind of cost savings is at variance with another. However, there really is no paradox: people are simply expected to respond to the increased "bargain" dental care represents by spending more on it. We might have reason to worry about whether "too much" is being spent on dentistry only if we suspect that people systematically misjudge the value of what they are buying.

THE ROLE OF INSURANCE

The standard, but by no means universally accepted, explanation of burgeoning health care expenditures has been the dramatic increase in third-party payment. By 1979 about 76 percent of the American people had some form of private hospitalization insurance, and public insurance paid the bills of so many other people that only 13 percent of payments for hospital care in 1980 were made directly by the consumer.[16] Those who stress demand factors to account for the increase of health care expenditures point to the physician propensity to do as much as possible for their patients, rather than engaging in even rudimentary cost-benefit analysis. When third party payment is available, physicians are largely or completely unrestrained in ordering whatever care they think is necessary.

For dental care there was very little insurance coverage until quite recently. As health insurance benefits were gained in the collective bargaining process, and as higher incomes raised the attractiveness of untaxed benefits, more and more workplace-based insurance developed. In 1960 only 2.3 percent of the U.S. civilian population had some kind of dental insurance; 30.2 percent had it by 1979.[17] It must be stressed, however, that unlike much health insurance, dental insurance still leaves its beneficiaries paying quite a substantial part of annual expenses. A typical Delta Dental (professionally sponsored) policy in the early '80s called for $25 to $50 in deductible payments per enrollee with 20 to 50 percent coinsurance for many services.[18] Commercial insurance policies are often similar and frequently employ even greater cost-sharing. Nonetheless, there is every reason to believe that the existence of insurance is substantially increasing the effective demand for dental services because dental care is quite responsive to price, and because insurance lowers the effective price of service.[19]

Jeffrey E. Harris has recently argued[20] that insurance-generated health expenditures may provide funds for the development of new treatment techniques and other medical advances that would otherwise be underproduced from the standpoint of society. This argument assumes that medical research would lag without the insurance-generated subsidies. No such argument can be made concerning dental research. Dentistry remains largely a "cottage industry," and there is no indication that any substantial part of the extra demand generated by dental insurance induces a more rapid rate of technological innovation in the dental-care system. More specifically, the only effective research and development in dentistry and dental health in general is done quite independently of patient revenues. In the absence of any significant impact from one person's consumption of dental care on the welfare of others, and in view of the fact that most people understand full well that their failure to take care of their teeth will cause discomfort and ultimately tooth loss, many analysts have found it hard to justify public support of consumption (at least for adults) above that which would be chosen by the typical person facing the full market price.[21]

DENTAL CARE AND PUBLIC POLICY

Several major government policies—implicit and explicit—have had important impacts on dental care markets. Understanding their history, present status, and probable future course can take us a long way toward forecasting the future of the entire dental care sector, including unit costs and total expenditures for dental services.

Since 1963, dental schools have been heavily subsidized by the federal government. Between 1965 and 1978 the capacity of the schools increased by 53 percent. This explains most of the dramatic increase in the dentist-population ratio in recent years. The ratio was 1 to 2,070 in 1965, 1 to 1,907 in 1975 and is projected to reach 1 to 1,612 by 1990.[22] In addition to supporting a permanent increase in the country's physical capacity to produce dentists, the federal government has been heavily subsidizing the process of dental education. During the seventies dental schools received up to three thousand dollars or more in federal operating subsidy per student. This support ended in 1981.[23] Some observers see the termination of federal assistance and the increasing number of dentists relative to the population as signals that the present number of dental school places cannot be sustained. At the time of this writing, however, there has been only a modest decrease in dental-school enrollment nationwide.

Historically, tacit immunity conferred by the major antitrust agencies on professionally sponsored anticompetitive activities has been another important area of public policy affecting dental care. Since *Goldfarb* v. *Virginia* in 1975,[24] however, that approval has been crumbling. The culmination came in 1977 with the Bates decision in which bar association bans on advertising by lawyers were made unenforceable. Two years later an agreement was reached between the American Dental Association and the Federal Trade Commission removing many professionally sponsored advertising restrictions. Most observers expect a dramatic increase in advertising by dentists in coming years.[25] From the standpoint of reducing dental care costs, it is clear that advertising should encourage price competition and reduce profits in dentistry by increasing the sensitivity of dentists to their markets. Advertising is likely to interact with dentist supply to put an unprecedented squeeze on dentist incomes despite a possibly growing demand resulting from increased insurance coverage and rising incomes.

Like most other professions, dentistry has been given considerable powers of self-regulation. The power to forbid advertising has now been largely removed from its purview. Control over who may provide dental services continues to reside with state dental boards.[26] There are now three main categories of personnel found in dental practices in addition to dentists and secretary-receptionists. The traditional dental assistant simply aids the dentist in administering services to the patient but performs few services independently. The dental hygienist performs prophylaxes (teeth cleaning), exposes and processes radiographs, applies fluoride solutions, and teaches dental hygiene. Dental technicians work in laboratories to fabricate artificial teeth and dentures.

The challenge to dentists from lesser-trained personnel is now apparent on at least three fronts. First, some dental hygienists have taken seriously the public's apparent distaste for government regulation and have established themselves as independent entrepreneurs, despite legal problems in all states.[27] Second, technicians in many states have established themselves as denturists, fitting people for false teeth. Some form of this practice is legal in eight of the ten Canadian provinces and in three states.[28] Finally, scores of tests in many countries have demonstrated that a very large fraction of all dental procedures can be performed by personnel called Expanded Function (or Duty) Dental Auxiliaries (EFDAs). These persons, with various kinds of training that seldom exceed two years of professional education—compared to the dentist's usual four—have been blocked in nearly all states from performing most duties beyond those of dental assistants, even under the supervision of a dentist.[29] Although widespread practice by EFDAs certainly could lower the cost of dental care very substantially, there is little prospect of a loosening of these restrictions. Foreign experience suggests that relaxation has occurred only under conditions of a perceived shortage of dentists; there is little reason to expect an exception in the United States.[30]

As we have seen, the exclusion of health benefits from taxable income for employees has played an important role in the growth of dental insurance. Economic theory and the experience elsewhere in the health care sector suggest that such insurance has increased both the unit price and the volume of dental services and hence total expenditures. Unsurprisingly, some policy analysts have long favored the removal of such tax advantages,[31] but the proposal seemed politically infeasible. During the past few years, however, there has been increasing attention to the possibility that consumers could be obliged to pay more attention to their health care expenditures by removing enough tax support for health insurance so that most people would be facing the entire price of insurance in the range where they actually make their insurance purchase decisions. The best known plan of this kind is Alain Enthoven's Consumer Choice Plan.[32] Its implications for dentistry seem unambiguous. Enthoven proposes to allow an insurance tax credit for an average income citizen of about 60 percent of the per capita expenditures for covered services in a given area. Certain features of qualifying insurance, including catastrophic coverage, are specified.

Enthoven's example of covered services is physician visits and hospital costs. He notes that: "A higher or lower amount based on a more or less extensive list of covered services and on broad political judgments about priorities, might be chosen as the basis for the subsidies."[33] The inclusion of dental services appears allowable under this phrasing but is most unlikely. There are two main reasons. First, dental health is unlikely to be considered a "priority." Second, a major purpose of the Enthoven plan is to reduce the insurance-induced consumption of health care services while avoiding serious hardship. It would be extremely difficult to make a case that the absence of dental care insurance would result in considerable hardship. Most dental treatment needs result from personal neglect; treatment costs are modest relative to most incomes, and treatment usually can be spread (and hence budgeted) over a considerable period of time if necessary.[34] In fact, dental insurance appears to be almost the ideal target for the cessation of all tax subsidy.

The result of the introduction of the Enthoven plan or one of the many other "procompetitive" plans considered by the ninety-eighth Congress is that dental insurance would have to be purchased at unsubsidized prices. When characteristics of dental care just enumerated are considered with the administrative costs of an insurance scheme, the tendency for insured persons to get more treatment than others, and the skewness of demand for dental care by those of upper incomes, even in the presence of insurance, it appears that the price of unsubsidized dental insurance policies would look unattractive to most consumers.[35]

A change in the tax status of health insurance is the most probable federal policy likely to affect substantially the total demand for dental services in the near future. Demand resulting from public programs is very unlikely to increase during the 1980s. Indeed, spending cuts are likely to reduce dental benefits. All levels of government spent only $600 million on dental services in 1980. Medicaid accounted for about $500 million. Most of the rest went to salaried dentists in government programs for specific groups.[36]

In the early 1970s it appeared that vastly increased public benefits for dentistry were likely because three of the leading health insurance bills included substantial dental benefits.[37] The Nixon-Ford CHIP plan would have provided dental benefits for those under thirteen years old with only 10 percent coinsurance for the poor, but with both a deductible and a coinsurance rate that rose steeply with income. The Democratic Kennedy-Mills bill offered a flat 25 percent coinsurance rate and no deductible for children, regardless of age or family income. The most complete major national health insurance plan, embodied in the Kennedy-Corman bill, would have provided immediate free coverage to all persons under eighteen years old with coverage for all persons under twenty-six years old added over the first five years of the plan's operation. Ultimately, it was envisioned that the entire population would be covered, although coverage for those over twenty-five years old might be limited to approved modes of services such as health maintenance organizations or prepaid non-profit plans. And all of the services would be "free;" the Kennedy-Corman plan did call for out-of-pocket payment.

When the Carter administration came to office in 1977 many thought that some kind of national health insurance was on the way. Yet by the second half of that administration it was very clear that the condition of the economy and the mood of the nation precluded any major new domestic spending programs. The outcome of the 1980 election placed national health insurance still lower on the list of likely federal initiatives. But national health insurance, with its strong support from organized labor and many other consumer and church groups, clearly will make its way to the top of the legislative agenda again. Some form of insurance for catastrophic illness may well come in the not-too-distant future. Such coverage has always had the support of conservatives principally as a way to defuse the entire national health insurance issue. For exactly this reason, liberals have not been anxious to enact catastrophic coverage alone. But times change. No major group would want to be portrayed as holding the American people hostage while awaiting a more complete insurance plan that might be feasible only much later. It is the combination of catastrophic coverage and the limitation of the tax credit that makes the Enthoven plan perhaps the only politically appealing new health insurance plan to be presented in a very long time. The impact of this plan on dentistry already has been discussed. Moreover, even if the political situation should change rapidly and more conventional national health insurance becomes a possibility, it is questionable whether dental benefits would be included. Government-financed coverage for children under age thirteen would have cost several billion dollars in the mid-1970s, while universal dental coverage would have cost at least $20 billion.[38] It is hard to imagine a political climate so drastically changed from the present one that such enormous expenditures would be borne to alleviate such modest perceived hardship.

THE BOOK THAT FOLLOWS

In a book of this length, it is not possible to deal with all of the ways in which cost savings in dentistry might be realized, but the several chapters do cover a broad range of approaches to the problem. In Chapter 1, Douglas Conrad and Peter Milgrom lay out some of the probable results of the increasing competitiveness in dental care markets. Advertising, franchising, multiple-dentist practices, and increased use of auxiliaries can, in their view, be expected to change the face of dentistry quite considerably over the coming years. Their paper particularly stresses the ways in which competition will tend to reduce prices relative to production costs and thus reduce "costs" for the consumer.

In Chapter 2, Howard Bailit and Robert Kudrle take a look at the various delivery systems that can be employed in dentistry. Prepaid group practices, provision of services by salaried government employees, and the role of school and work-place-based delivery are explored. This chapter, more than Chapter 1, stresses the potential of different delivery systems for lowering the real production costs of dental services.

Chapter 3 takes the question of reducing production costs one step farther. David Born explores the cost-reducing potential of utilizing people with lesser training than dentists in the independent fitting and manufacture of dentures and the provision of dental hygiene services. He also provides an interpretation of dentistry's historical ambivalence toward the most-explored cost-reduction measure of all: the employment of Expanded Duty Dental Auxiliaries.

The training of dentists is extraordinarily expensive. Furthermore, federal support for dental education is being cut back. Sheldon Rovin, Richard Scheffler, and Jeffrey Bauer present a critical look at the state of dental education in Chapter 4. They explore opportunities for dental education to become more efficient and more relevant to the needs of a changing professional environment. The chapter also offers suggestions about how dental education could generate more patient revenue.

The American people evidence widely varying attitudes towards dental care and widely varying contact with the dental care system. Each pattern of contact—preventative, intermittent, or only as a response to serious symptoms—generates an expected level of out-of-pocket costs. Choosing a sensible pattern of care represents a potentially important form of cost saving by individuals. In Chapter 5, Kenneth Warner and Brian Burt explore these cost patterns systematically through computer simulation.

The dentist has considerable latitude in the kind of treatment chosen for a specific problem. Beyond this, there is additional discretion in the skill and care taken in the performance of the ensuing procedures. Individuals, private third-party payers and government agencies all have an interest in effective monitoring of the quality of dental care. In Chapter 6 Marvin Marcus and Samuel Tobin explore the options available under a quality assurance system.

In the final chapter of the book, the editors summarize the contents of the preceding chapters and suggest future research needs.

Notes

1. Material in this and the following three paragraphs is drawn from Robert T. Kudrle, "Dental Care," Chapter 12 in Judith Feder, John Holahan, and Theodore Marmor, eds., *National Health Insurance: Conflicting Goals and Policy Choices*, (Washington: The Urban Institute, 1980).

2. See, for example, Victor Fuchs, *Who Shall Live?*, (New York: Basic Books, Inc., 1975), Chapter 1; M. Kenneth Bowler, Robert T. Kudrle, and Theodore Marmor, "The Political Economy of National Health Insurance: Policy Analysis and Political Evaluation," in Kenneth M. Friedman and Stuart H. Rakoff, eds., *Toward a National Health Policy* (Lexington, Mass.: D. C. Heath and Company, 1977).

3. Kudrle, "Dental Care," p. 576.

4. Preston, Littleton, Jr. "Differences Between the Medical and Dental Health Care Sectors," in Jesse Hixon, ed., *The Target Income Hypothesis and Related Issues in Health Manpower* (Washington: Division of Dentistry, DHEW publication no. HRA 80-27), p. 201.

5. L. Benham, A. Maurizi, and M. W. Reder, "Migration, Location, and Remuneration of Medical Personnel: Physicians and Dentists," *Review of Economics and Statistics*, 50 (August, 1968), p. 338.

6. Kudrle, "Dental Care," p. 576.

7. Ibid., p. 579.

8. Warren Greenberg, "Provider-Influenced Insurance Plans and Their Impact on Competition: Lessons from Dentistry," 1980, mimeographed.

9. U.S. Department of Health, Education and Welfare, Advisory Committee and Dental Health to the Secretary, *Report and Recommendations* (Washington, D.C.: U.S. Government Printing Office, 1973), p. 21.

10. Information in this and the following paragraph is drawn from Robert M. Gibson and Daniel R. Waldo, "National Health Expenditures, 1980," *Health Care Financing Review* 3(1):1-54, 1980. Kudrle, "Dental Care," p. 579 and pp. 604-605.

11. Kudrle, "Dental Care," p. 579 and pp. 604-605.

12. H. L. Bailit, M. Raskin, S. Reisine, and D. Chiriboga, "Controlling the Cost of Dental Care," *American Journal of Public Health*, 69(7):699-703, 1979.

13. *Statistical Abstract of the United States* (Washington, D.C.: U.S. Government Printing Office, 1980).

14. The index is an unweighted average of only four services.

15. Alex Maurizi, "Rates of Return to Dentistry and the Decision to Enter Dental School," *Journal of Human Resources* 10 (Fall, 1975), pp. 521-28; Stephen T. Mennemeyer, "Really Great Returns to Medical Education?" *Journal of Human Resources* 13 (Winter, 1978), pp. 75-90. See also the discussion in Chapter 4 of this book.

16. Marjorie Smith Carroll and Ross H. Arnett III, "Private Health Insurance Plans in 1978 and 1979: A Review of Coverage, Enrollment, and Financial Experience," *Health Care Financing Review*, September 1981, p. 56. Gibson and Waldo, "National Health Expenditures, 1980," p. 21.

17. Carroll and Arnett, "Private Health Insurance Plans," pp. 16 and 18; the earlier fig-

ure is for gross enrollment, but few persons were eligible for multiple coverage at that time.

18. Information provided by Delta Dental Plan of Minnesota.

19. See Willard G. Manning and Charles E. Phelps, *Dental Care Demand: Point Estimates and Implications for National Health Insurance* (Santa Monica: The Rand Corporation, 1978).

20. An accessible source of some of these ideas is Jeffrey E. Harris, "Commentary," in Mark V. Pauly, ed., *National Health Insurance: What Now, What Later, What Never?* (Washington: American Enterprise Institute, 1980), pp. 264-269.

21. See, for example, Robert G. Evans and M. F. Williamson, *Extending Canadian Health Insurance: Options for Pharmacare and Denticare* (Toronto: University of Toronto Press, 1978), p. 125.

22. James Ake, *Dental Manpower Fact Book*, (Washington: U.S. D.H.E.W., 1979), pp. 43-62.

23. Information provided by Dr. Jeffrey Bauer of the University of Colorado School of Dentistry.

24. For an excellent discussion of the issue, see Clark C. Havighurst, "Antitrust Enforcement in the Medical Services Industry: What Does It All Mean?" *Milbank Memorial Fund Quarterly, Health and Society*, vol. 58, no. 1 (1980), pp. 89-124.

25. See discussion in Chapter 1.

26. For an exhaustive discussion, see Owen McBride, "Restrictive Licensing of Dental Paraprofessionals," *The Yale Law Journal*, 83 (1974), pp. 802-826.

27. See discussion in Chapter 1.

28. See discussion in Chapter 3.

29. See McBride, "Restrictive Licensing."

30. Robert T. Kudrle, "The Implications of Foreign Dental Coverage for U.S. National Health Insurance," *Journal of Health Politics, Policy and Law*, Winter 1981.

31. The best-known argument is Martin S. Feldstein, "A New Approach to National Health Insurance," *The Public Interest*, 23 (Spring 1971).

32. Alain C. Enthoven, *Health Plan*, (Reading, Mass.: Addison-Wesley Publishing Co., 1980).

33. Ibid., p. 120.

34. For a similar argument with data about actual expenditures, see Kudrle, "Dental Care," p. 570.

35. For a concrete example of this issue drawn from medical care, see Feldstein, "A New Approach."

36. Gibson, "National Health Expenditures, 1980," p. 42.

37. Kudrle, "Dental Benefits," pp. 581-609.

38. For a simple estimate of costs, see Robert T. Kudrle, "Dental Coverage Under National Health Insurance," report prepared for the Robert Wood Johnson Foundation under Grant No. 2505, 1977, mimeographed.

Reducing the Cost of Dental Care

1

Market Forces

Douglas A. Conrad and Peter Milgrom

INTRODUCTION

This chapter will analyze the role of market forces in containing dental-care costs. "Market forces" are the whole range of supply, demand, and structural factors that shape the dental-care market. In analyzing the role of these forces, this paper will examine how supply, demand, and the market structure in which dental services are delivered interact with one another to determine dental-care costs.

Several developments promise to affect dental costs significantly during the eighties. These include market developments in the private sector, social and demographic changes, and initiatives in the public sphere (such as price controls, antitrust actions, and state regulatory and legislative changes). Private market forces include the broadening use of prepaid dental plans; rising input costs, particularly the increasing costs of precious metals; the growth of alternative dental delivery systems; altering patterns of market competition, and changing trends in the relative mix of dentists and auxiliary personnel in the dental profession. Socio-demographic shifts that will alter the type and volume of dental services demanded in the future include changes in the age distribution, education, and personal income of the United States population. Finally, public initiatives that are mapping new directions in the dental-care market include the Federal Trade Commission's

Research for this paper was supported by Contract No. 232-78-0188 from the Health Resources Administration and Grant Nos. HS-01978 and HS-03603 from the National Center for Health Services Research.

Robert O'Shea and David Striffler provided helpful comments on the original draft of this chapter.

(FTC) interim consent agreement with the American Dental Association (ADA) concerning dental advertising[1] and the Council of State
Governments' publication[2] of a model state dental-practice act.

Market forces for cost containment, including supply-side and
demand-side factors plus the extent of market competition, are high-
lighted in Table 1. The factors influence dental-care costs by affecting
both the unit costs of dental services (technical efficiency) and the
relationship between the prices charged and the costs of those services
(allocative efficiency). For example, rising input costs for energy and
precious metals will contribute to increased unit costs of dental services, whereas state dental practice act and professional restrictions
will affect primarily the nature and extent of competition among
providers in local dental-care markets.

Table 1. Cost Containment Factors

Factors	Influence on Cost through	
	Technical Efficiency	Allocative Efficiency
Supply-side		
State dental practice and limits on:		
ownership form	X	X
number of offices		X
auxiliaries per dentist	X	X
extent of task delegation to auxiliaries	X	X
interstate reciprocity of licensure		X
independent practice of dental hygiene		X
Evolution in the form and size of dental practices	X	X
Macroeconomic activity	X	X
Input price effects	X	
Demand-side		
Growth of prepaid dental plans	X	X
Changing patterns of advertising activity in the dental care marketplace	X	X

On the supply side, this analysis pinpoints four key factors: state
dental-practice act restrictions, the changing number and mix of dental practitioners, the influence of macroeconomic activity, and the
effects of input prices on dental care. In many instances, these supply factors not only affect unit costs; because of their impact on
technical efficiency, they also can be expected to influence competition among dental-care providers.

Competition in dentistry is likely to be spurred by a minority of providers—those who achieve production economies by increasing practice size and using auxiliaries in cost-effective ways, and then pass these cost savings on to consumers via lower prices for dental services. As increased competition leads to reductions in the price-cost margins for dental services, prices in the dental market become more accurate signals of the actual costs of services.

In principle, improvements in this signaling function of prices lead to increased efficiency in the allocation of resources to dentistry (by matching the value of dental services to consumers with the cost of dental services. The eighties will offer an opportunity to test empirically, through a natural market experiment, the degree to which competitive forces can produce gains in allocative efficiency in the dental marketplace.

Macroeconomic activity will exert an important influence on the supply-side conditions of the dental market, in the eighties, mainly through the feedback effects of economy-wide demand on the income prospects of dentists. The demand for dental services and the net income of dentists is highly sensitive to movements in the aggregate economy. These demand-side factors influence competition and allocative efficiency within the dental market in several ways. For example, recession-induced declines in dentists' net incomes lead to pressures to reduce the supply of new practitioners and to restrain competitive forces that might further erode net incomes.

On the demand side, advertising activity and the growth of prepaid dental plans are the principal market forces governing dental-care costs. These factors reinforce the argument presented for the demand side: market forces generate feedback effects between technical and allocative efficiency. That is, allocative effects on competitive behavior and pricing in dentistry also create incentives for increased technical efficiency, and vice versa. For example, as the population covered by dental prepayment plan increases and as these plans become more comprehensive, the dimensions on which dentists might compete for patients shift away from price and toward amenities, convenience, and reductions in treatment time. At the same time, to the extent that large prepaid plans have sufficient leverage to enforce limits on maximum prices for dental services, dental practices are encouraged to minimize production costs (as a way to maximize net income subject to the price constraint). Advertising is expected to affect primarily allocative efficiency and the type and degree of market competition, but it also promotes productive efficiency.

SUPPLY-SIDE FACTORS IN DENTISTRY

Supply-side factors in dentistry include various manpower trends, independent practice of dental hygiene, the evolution of group and large-scale practices, and changes in state dental practice acts.

Manpower Trends

The econometric model of the Health Resources Administration[3] forecasts a gradual substitution of dentists' time for that of auxiliaries (hygienists, assistants, and clerical workers) over the period 1978-1995. Underlying this prediction is the assumption that the value of the dentist's own time will decline relative to the wage rates for auxiliaries. The authors posit that increasing competition in the dental care market will cause this reduction in the implicit relative price of the dentist's own time. The dentist-to-population ratio is forecasted to increase by 10.4 percent over the next decade,[4] and further competitive pressure is expected from dental advertising and non-traditional practices such as those of denturists and independent dental hygienists.[5] For several reasons, the HRA forecast seems to overstate the relative shift away from auxiliary employment. First of all, schools are likely to reduce their enrollment in response to declines in the federal subsidies for dental students, thereby controlling growth in the supply of new dentists. Second, the major opportunity for efficient practice during the eighties is still expected to be the increased use of modern techniques such as four-handed sit-down dentistry, which requires the assistance of trained auxiliaries. Moreover, the eighties will be the first decade in which a majority of dentists have received specific dental school training in the use of auxiliaries. This suggests more, not less, use of auxiliaries. Finally, the proportion of dental firms with more than one dentist is increasing,[6] and such firms typically employ a larger number of auxiliaries. Survey data[7] from 1976 suggest that practices with a greater number of auxiliaries are more profitable,[8] and that output expansion under competitive conditions is likely to be concentrated among these auxiliary-intensive practices. Competitive pressures will induce the dentist to search for more profitable[9] practice arrangements. This incentive should offset partially the effects of rising input prices for auxiliaries relative to dentist's own time.

In sum, existing economic data suggest that auxiliary-intensive practice will continue to be a reasonable strategy for cost containment for the dentist who responds to the competitive environment.

Independent Practice of Dental Hygiene

Recent developments in California, Kansas, and Pennsylvania[10] reflect increasing interest in and market experimentation with various forms of independent practice by dental hygienists. In Kingston, Pennsylvania, Susan Edwards, a licensed dental hygienist, opened her own practice to perform oral prophylaxes, defying state regulations that required hygienists to work under a dentist's supervision. In Kansas and California a few hygienists have been allowed to function as "independent contractors." As an independent contractor, the hygienist enters into a compromise agreement with a dentist who sends patients for prophylaxis to the hygienist; the hygienist typically works in an adjacent office under the loose supervision of the dentist. The independent contractors in these cases determine and collect their own fees and pay their own practice expenses. Either of these independent practice models is likely to place downward pressure on prevailing fees for prophylaxis, oral hygiene instruction, and the administration of topical fluorides.

The downward pressure on prices comes from competition among dentists and independent hygienists in the market for these preventive services and from reduced unit costs for performing such services, where the hygienist-entrepreneur requires a smaller absolute return on human capital and where the investment in physical capital is considerably less. The training costs of hygienists and their alternative opportunities are less than those of dentists, which implies that hygienists will offer their human capital to the market for less. A study of the costs of restorative services for the Forsyth Clinic, staffed by teams of advanced-skills hygienists and dental assistants under a dentist's supervision, estimated potential savings of 44 percent in the Forsyth model relative to prevailing dental fees for restorative services.[11] Since the relative advantage of having a dentist perform restorative services is greater than that of having a dentist perform preventive procedures, the Forsyth study seems to yield at least an approximation of the proportionate price reductions one can expect from independent hygiene practice focused on traditional preventive procedures.

If independent-dental hygiene practices are to operate efficiently and successfully, they must be suitably located. One possible setting for practices would be in high-volume retail stores, where large numbers of consumers can be easily attracted to the practice. It should also be noted that such delivery models might have the indirect effect of drawing new patients into the market for professional dental care.

The independent practice of hygiene could provide a kind of "institutional advertising" for dentistry as a whole.

Evolution of Group and Large-Scale Practices

Recent econometric evidence[12] indicates increasing returns owing to increasing dental practice size. Practices with three and four or more dentists are estimated to produce 8 and 22 percent more visits than two-dentist practices.

These findings are reinforced by the trend toward larger practices in dentistry. According to the yearly *Survey of Dental Practice* by the American Dental Association, the size distribution of firms is tilting in the direction of multi-dentist practices and toward a larger scale of practice. Underlying differences in net-income prospects support the continuation of these trends. For example, the 1976 survey found that the median net income for a single dentist in practice with three operatories, one assistant, one secretary, and one hygienist equaled $41,501, as compared to $71,958 for a single dentist in practice with five operatories and six or more auxiliaries.

A recent study by the Research Triangle Institute (RTI) also compared group practices of varying size with solo dental practices.[13] Using gross billings adjusted for fee differences among dentists as the measure of annual output, the RTI findings were similar to those of Kushman et al.:[14] three- or four-dentist practices and five-dentist practices were 19.2 percent and 25.1 percent more productive than two-dentist practices. No significant differences were observed between solo and two-dentist practices. Douglass and Day[15] cite early results from the RTI analysis that suggest that solo-practice may deliver proportionately more primary-care dental services, e.g., preventive and basic corrective services. Further analysis is required to discern the reasons for these apparent differences. Thus, while the evidence is ambiguous, it does seem to suggest that increased practice size is one way to improve the technical efficiency of dentistry.

Group practices also confront an incentive problem. If revenues are shared among dentists in the group, payment methods must be devised to maintain the individual dentist's incentive to produce. The individual incentive to produce must be balanced with the functioning of the group as a team and with the administrative costs of identifying individual output within a team production process (in, for example, cases of within-group referrals and consultation). Interestingly, Kushman et al.[16] reported that dentists in practices that shared revenue were less productive for a given level of inputs than those in which each dentist retained [his or her] own earnings. It was not clear from the data whether the differences were attributable to managerial inefficiency or preferences for a more leisurely work pace.

Changes in State Dental-Practice Acts

State dental-practice acts influence several dimensions of the dental market, including entry conditions to local areas, the nature and scale of individual dental practices, the type and level of auxiliary employment for individual practices, the degree of market competition, and the aspects of dental services (e.g., price, "quality", convenience) in which competition takes place. Four types of practice act provisions are discussed below: reciprocal dental licensing agreements among states, limits on the number of offices that may be owned and operated by a single dentist, limits on the number of hygienists (and, in one state, auxiliaries) per dentist, prohibitions against nondentist ownership of dental practices, and prohibitions against the use of trade names by dental practices. These provisions affect the individual dentist's technical efficiency, as well as the allocative efficiency of the dental care system as a whole.

Interstate reciprocity of dental licensure. Over the period 1970-76, the number of states without reciprocal licensing agreements for dentists declined from 35 to 18, according to the *American Dental Directory*.[17] Several studies shed light on the effects of the absence of reciprocity on dental prices. Shepard's empirical analysis of 1970 ADA data[18] revealed that prices (based on a composite of fees for 12 dental services) were about 14.9 percent higher in states without reciprocity agreements. House's work with 1976 American Dental Association data[19] suggested that the absence of reciprocity was associated with a 5.1 to 6.6 percent increase in a composite index of dental prices. It should be noted that both studies yield estimates of the supply-side response to reciprocity limits. On the demand side, a 5 percent rise in price will lead to approximately a 7.5 percent reduction in the quantity of dental visits (based on a price elasticity of demand of -1.5, which is well within the range of most available estimates).[20]

Limits of reciprocity act as barriers to the interstate mobility of dental practitioners. Such barriers potentially cut two ways: limits on reciprocity reduce inflows to states that would otherwise experience net in-migration (i.e., those with unimpeded interstate mobility of dentists) and reduce outflows for states that would otherwise have net out-migration. Therefore, the a priori effect of the absence of reciprocity on dental prices in a particular state is indeterminate. However, the empirical studies do suggest that, on balance, the absence of reciprocity does contribute to a smaller stock of dentists within the nonreciprocity states[21] and thus to higher dental prices[22] in those states. One empirical analysis finds that limits on reciprocity exert their most statistically significant and largest effects on certain expensive "specialty" services, e.g., root canals, bridges, and gold crowns.[23] This is consistent with Littleton's hypothesis[24] that reciprocity limits are a differential barrier to specialists.

One approach to enhancing dentists' interstate mobility is examination by regional dental testing boards (RDTB). Regional testing, in which individual states delegate responsibility for clinical examination to a separate body, departs from the historical pattern of individual state-specific clinical testing. Successful completion of the regional board's exam meets the clinical requirement for licensure in each member state. As of January 1979, 33 states plus the District of Columbia were included in four regional boards,[25] the first regional exam having been conducted in 1969. In their preliminary study of the effect of such RDTBs, Budner and Goldman did not find any measurable impact of the boards on the distribution of dentists, mobility of established practitioners, or on the choice of initial practice location. Apart from difficulties with the data base and lack of controls on other variables influencing dentists' mobility patterns (which were acknowledged), the authors explained their findings by noting that the regional testing boards were not created to improve dental manpower distribution. In their judgment, specific regional problems, such as lack of multiple licensure for the single market area overlapping suburban Maryland, Virginia, and the District of Columbia, seem to have provided the major impetus for RDTBs. In the absence of an analysis that controls for other factors influencing dentists' location decisions, it appears that one cannot yet judge how RDTBs have affected manpower distribution and dental prices.

Limits on number of offices. A June 1980[26] analysis revealed that dental-practice acts of five states presently incorporate specific limitations on the opening of more than one office: the limit on the number of "satellite" offices is one in California and two in Texas, Iowa, Kentucky, and Connecticut. An analysis of state-practice acts[27] suggests there will be a gradual removal of these restrictions. A related *Dental Management* survey[28] found that 8.3 percent of respondents from various regions of the country were practicing in more than one office.

In the same study, detailed case histories of nine practitioners operating satellite offices pointed to the following patterns:

Most satellite offices were acquired through the purchase of an existing practice.

Most dentists divided their time equally between the satellite and the primary office, as did their associate dentists.

The increase in income attributed to the operation of the satellite office ranged from 20 to 100 percent. Satellite offices begun from scratch took appreciably longer to pay for themselves than did established practices that were purchased. This seems to suggest that certain intangible assets, such as the good will developed in established practices, is transferable in the market for dental practices.

In its recently published model, state dental-practice act,[29] the Council of State Governments challenged the rationale for statutory limits on the number of dental offices by arguing that the rules had little apparent relation to protecting public health and safety. Moreover, testimony in the case of *Gilmartin* v. *California Board of Dental Examiners* suggests that the principal objective of the two-office rule in California was to block the growth of chain-operated, advertising dental practices, not to prevent moderated expansion of private practices.

Rules regulating the number of offices per practice also hamper arrangements by which a single dentist could supply capital for several offices and maintain ownership interest in each. As the financial risk-bearer for each office, the dentist-owner could promote the decentralized practice of dentistry in several locations. A single dentist entrepreneur might lease office space and dental equipment to other dentists in return for a share in the net income of each practice. This argument does not assume imperfection in the capital market, but implies instead that a limit on number of offices reduces the efficiency of entrepreneurial risk-taking. The entrepreneurial input, not financial capital per se, is the constrained resource in this case. The potential income-sharing arrangements between the lessor and the other dentists could range from payment of salaries by the lessor, to profit-sharing among the lessor and other dentists.

In sum, limits on the number of offices can be expected to hinder the development of multi-dentist networks of practices. Similar legal provisions also restrict the use of multiple locations by a single dentist, although the time constraints and logistical difficulties of a single dentist practicing in more than two or three locations would limit such arrangements anyway. Finally, limited-office rules also restrict the practice arrangements open to newly graduated dentists.

The new dentist may not wish to bear the risk of full ownership of a practice but would be willing to become established as an associate of a primary dentist who acts as the entrepreneur. By foreclosing such options, limited-office rules implicitly raise the costs of entry into dental-care markets.

An analysis of 1971 data on dental-service prices in 39 standard metropolitan statistical areas (SMSAs), controlled for certain supply, demand, and legal factors, and adjusted for cross-sectional differences in cost of living, suggested that average dental fees were approximately four percent higher in SMSAs within states having limits on the number of offices.[30] One should be cautious about the finding, however, because it is based on scanty data and there is little known about the economic mechanism involved in this problem.

Nondentist ownership and use of trade names. The ownership of practices by other than licensed dentists is generally prohibited by state dental-practice acts, as is the use of trade names by dental practices. However, the development of corporate franchising of dental practices is eroding the margins of statutory restraints. Two current corporate models illustrate this trend. In cooperation with Montgomery Ward and Co., a nationwide corporation, Dent Care Systems Ltd., is opening dental practices in department store locations. In California, Montgomery Ward receives a share of the earnings of each dentist franchise.[31]

The Peoples Drug Store chain plans to be the first in the nation to put dentists in its drug stores. The first two clinics are scheduled to open in Maryland and the District of Columbia. The offices will be owned and operated by a Maryland dentist to comply with state laws prohibiting nondentist ownership. The owner-dentist will not practice in the offices, but will hire five other dentists to work for him. Family Dental Centers, a company that includes the dentist and two nondentist partners, will operate and finance the clinics.[32]

These two examples highlight how franchising arrangements have adjusted to state laws. To the extent that ownership is defined as a claim to the profits of an enterprise, the effective ownership of dental practices is broadened subtly by the introduction of corporate franchising. Perhaps even more important, current dental advertising makes frequent and explicit use of trade names. For example, a newspaper advertisement reprinted in *The Advertising Dentist* clearly links the Sterling Dental Center in Landover Hills, Maryland, with Sterling Optical, "a name you've known and trusted for over 20 years."[33]

The future of such practices will determine partially the growth of advertising and large dental practices. These forms of marketing and practice innovation have diffused more broadly and been adapted more rapidly among the "retail dental practices," as they often are called. Corporate financing arrangements and the ready availability of facilities can ease the transition to large-scale dental practice, so a growing partnership between dentists and the corporate sector seems likely. The cost-containment implications of these developments are uncertain, given the novelty of franchising arrangements. To the extent that they encourage auxiliary-intensive and large-scale dental practices, however, they suggest opportunities for improved technical and allocative efficiencies.

Limits on the number of hygienists per dentist. Currently 12 states and the District of Columbia limit the number of hygienists that a licensed dentist may employ. When these constraints are binding on dental practice organization, they act as a kind of tax on hygienists. Because the legal limits "tax" the *number* of hygienists but not the hygienists' duties or hours of work, one would predict:

Fewer hygienists per dentist

More hours worked per hygienist

Expansion of the functions performed by each of the smaller number of hygienists employed

Reduction in output, owing to the external constraint on input choices.

The net effect of these adjustments would be an increase in the cost of dental services.

Although economic theory would suggest testable hypotheses if limits on the number of hygienists per dentist represent binding constraints, it is very likely that these legal barriers only restrain dentists in group practices characterized by significant use of hygienists. Consequently, limits on the number of hygienists per dentist may create a particular barrier to group practice.

Existing empirical studies do not address the differential effect of hygienist limits on group dental practices. However, the studies highlight interesting findings: other things being equal, higher auxiliary wages are observed in states with such limits,[34] and the process of input substitution differs between states with and without these restrictions.[35] In restrictive states, auxiliaries are complementary to the dentist's time. Increased output is achieved primarily by increasing the dentist's working hours and the number of operatories. Conversely, in nonrestrictive states, auxiliaries substitute for the dentist. Output is increased by hiring auxiliaries, resulting in smaller increases in dentist working hours. One study,[36] based on 1971 SMSA data, suggests that average dental prices are about 4 percent higher in metropolitan areas with these constraints, other things being equal. A related analysis of state data from 1970 found that hygienist limits had a strong positive effect on fees for oral prophylaxis (a service performed predominantly by hygienists), as one would expect if the limits on the number of hygienists were constituting a truly binding constraint on production.

The "Target-Income" Hypothesis

The principal basis for interest in the "target-income" hypothesis is the positive correlation between provider/population ratios and provider fees reported in certain cross-sectional empirical studies. The "strong" form of the target-income model says that individual dentists increase discretionary demand for their services to offset external influence on their net-income prospects. Thus, the dentist, acting as the patient's agent, tends to set fees and adjust the patient's demand to maintain a "target" level of net income. The mechanism the dentist supposedly uses to determine target income has never been spelled out. The decision to recommend treatment for any one problem is highly discretionary, however, so the idea that the dentist could induce some demand for services is not beyond the realm of possibility. Accordingly, and in the absence of an explanation for how the target is set, proponents of this model generally assert a weak form of the hypothesis in which a certain degree of demand creation is possible.

One version of the model, as interpreted by Sloan and Feldman,[37] assumes that the dentist seeks to maximize utility, which is related positively to net income, negatively to the dentist's own time input, and negatively to the degree of demand creation. In other words, the dentist does not like to create demand, since doing so subtracts from leisure time, even though economic benefits result. In this form of the target-income model, an exogenous shock, such as an increase in the supply of dental practitioners in the locality, will initially drive down net income per practice. This will induce dentists to prescribe more services and raise prices until the marginal loss of utility due to demand creation (which is assumed to increase with net income) and forgone leisure is balanced by the marginal utility of the net income gained by such actions.

Empirical evidence and certain structural features of the dental-care market do not support the target-income hypothesis. First,

Shepard's work[38] found a negative association between dentist supply and dentist fees, a result consistent with the conventional economic model. Further, the experience of the Economic Stabilization Program provides a persuasive counterexample.[39] During 1970-72, a period generally without wage and price controls, dentists' real incomes increased 3.8 percent per year. During the control period (approximately 1972-74) dentists' real incomes declined by 10.1 percent per year. During the "catch-up" period of 1974-76 dentists' real incomes increased 3.5 percent per year—an increase below that of the pre-controls period and hardly indicative of the compensatory increase the target-income model would predict. Also, the difference between the composite index of dental prices and the index of average dental costs during the controlled period would imply only a 2 percent decline in real income. The difference of 8.1 percent (10.1 percent minus 2.0 percent) approximates the decline in utilization per dentist. If the target-income model is to be useful for prediction, it would have to explain why compensatory demand (utilization) creation was not more successful during the 1972-74 period.

In addition, the price elasticity of demand for dental services is high enough to hint that consumers respond to price signals in the dental market. This price sensitivity implies a sensitivity to total out-of-pocket cost, which places definite limits on demand creation by providers. As a related point, empirical studies of the extent of competition in dentistry have not rejected the competitive model.[40] By promoting the availability of alternatives, competition among providers will control demand creation.

A recent study directly addresses the issue of target-income behavior in dentistry. Musgrave[41] used 1976 price and utilization data from the Health Insurance Association of America (HIAA) to estimate a three-equation model of the supply of dental services, demand for dental services, and the dentist/population ratio. His study improves on most of the empirical literature about the target-income hypothesis by modeling supply, demand and dentist density simultaneously. Thus, his estimates permit the disentanglement of price effects caused by provider demand-creation from price effects caused by exogenous shifts in market supply and demand.[42]

Musgrave tested the supply-induced demand (or target income) hypothesis by including dentist density as an explanatory variable in the demand equation. Musgrave observed a positive coefficient for dentist density, but because of substantial inconsistencies[43] between the overall results and previous work he concluded that "the results from the demand and supply equations lend little support to the supply-induced demand hypothesis."[44] However, the limitations of Musgrave's data[45] warrant caution before rejecting the target-income hypothesis *solely* on the strength of his findings.

Manning and Phelps[46] present evidence to support an alternative explanation of the cross-sectional correlation between dentist density and dental fees. They estimated the effect of dentist density on demand for dental services among adult males compared to adult females.

The researchers found the effect of dentist density on utilization was more positive among adult males than among females. Given the higher value of missed work time for adult males (as estimated in the economic literature), the researchers interpreted their findings to mean that at least part of the effect of dentist density on demand is due to reduced time costs. House's work[47] suggests a similar interpretation.

On balance, the data do not appear to support the target-income hypothesis as a predictor of dentist behavior. This suggests that an increase in the supply of dental practitioners is likely to moderate the full price (the sum of the fee and implicit costs of patient time) of dental services.

ECONOMIC CONDITIONS AND DENTAL COSTS

Macroeconomic influences on dental-care costs include general U.S. economic conditions and energy costs. The literature documents a relatively high income elasticity (increase in demand owing to increases in consumer income) for dental care. The Rand Corporation estimates of income elasticity, for example, are .16 and .87 for white adult males and children respectively.[48]

House's recent time-series analysis[49] of dentists' incomes, fees, and practice costs during the 1952-1976 period provides further evidence of the sensitivity of the dental market to economic conditions. House's estimating equation[50] implied that a one percent increase in the rate of change in real GNP (Gross National Product in constant dollars) is associated with a 75 percent increase in the rate of change in dentists' real incomes. During the 1971-74 period of the economic stabilization program, which included the joint effects of recession and wage and price controls, dentist incomes declined at the precipitous rate of 10.1 percent per year.

An earlier American Dental Association (ADA) study of the period 1967-1975[51] showed dentists' fees tracking the movement of the Consumer Price Index—a 61.9 percent increase in dentists' fees was accompanied by a 61.2 percent rise in the Consumer Price Index.

The ADA study also documented significantly rising input costs during 1970-1975: prices of dentists' hand instruments such as amalgam carvers increased about 100 percent, endodontic files 60 percent, forceps 55 percent, prophylaxis angles more than 50 percent, and alloy about 100 percent. Meanwhile, it is clear that market forces such as the elasticity[52] of demand and inter-firm competition have limited the extent to which input cost increases have been passed on to consumers. Competition in the dental sector is likely to increase in the near future, and thus an even more marked continuation of these patterns is expected.

Energy costs. Rising energy costs are expected to affect the dental-delivery system. Energy costs increase the costs of travel to dental offices, thus increasing the importance of locational convenience to consumers. The relative importance of this factor is augmented by the growth in the breadth and depth of insurance that covers dental fees but not the "implicit" costs of dental care (such as travel). By placing a premium on geographic convenience, rising energy costs will to some degree reshape the geographic distribution of dental practices. For example, in the short run, the dental practice that draws from a wide geographic area can be expected to lose patients relative to competing practices whose patient population is more concentrated. Another effect in the short run will be to reduce specialization in the service mix of dentists whose clients are dispersed to the extent the service mix depends on economies of scale.

In the long run one would expect decreases in the fees of dentists with locational disadvantages and the relocation of dental practices to areas of more concentrated population. Multiple appointments for a dental procedure will be reduced, where possible, and a modest decline in their contribution to practice profitability should ensue (since their relative full cost to the consumer would increase, but the net return to the dentist has not). Finally, centralization (relative to population) of group dental practices including multiple specialties and general practitioners will increase, since these organizational forms minimize the travel costs of going to the referred dentist and permit individual practitioners to locate at jointly optimal points, allowing full realization of the economies of scale crucial to specialized practice.

DEMAND FORCES IN THE DENTAL CARE MARKET

Advertising and prepaid dental plans are the main issues affecting the demand side of the dental economy. As one examines the demand side, one also observes feedback effects on the supply side and on the extent and nature of market competition.

Advertising

In January 1977 the Federal Trade Commission (FTC) filed a formal complaint against the American Dental Association (ADA) and four of its component and constituent societies. The complaint alleged that through the enforcement of various sections of the ADA *Principles of Ethics*—primarily those pertaining to advertising and the soliciting of patients—the ADA and its societies had effectively fixed prices, hindered competition among dentists, restricted information of value to consumers, and hampered the development of innovative dental delivery systems.

In October 1977 the ADA House of Delegates passed a resolution advising local societies not to impose sanctions on member dentists who advertised. This action followed the Supreme Court ruling in *Bates* v. *State Bar of Arizona*[53] that bans on advertising of legal services are unconstitutional, in that restraints on advertising violated First Amendment guarantees of free speech. In addition, the ADA House of Delegates in 1977 approved guidelines for the definition of routine dental services for purposes of dentist advertising.[54] Essentially, the guidelines characterize as "routine" a service (1) performed frequently in the dental practice; (2) usually provided at a set fee; (3) provided with little or no variance in technique; and (4) including all professionally recognized components within generally accepted standards.

Legislatures and state dental boards are responding to these events by changing their rules and regulations on dental advertising. For example, recent revisions by the Missouri Dental Board[55] track the *Bates* decision quite closely.[56] The Missouri board's proscription on the use of electronic media may not prevail as the legal norm in the long term, however, since market forces—in particular, the cost-effectiveness of television and radio in reaching target audiences for dental advertising—are likely to overcome such rules.

On April 29, 1979, the ADA announced that the FTC had provisionally accepted a proposed settlement of the complaint against the ADA. Under terms of the interim settlement, the ADA agreed not to restrict or declare unethical and truthful advertising by dentists. Pending the outcome of the FTC complaint against the American Medical Association involving similar legal issues, the ADA and its societies would be permitted to impose sanctions only against members whose advertising is "false and misleading in any material respect."[57]

The result of this relaxation of ethical code and statutory restraints sets the stage for more extensive dentist advertising.

Advertising as Information. According to the "advertising as information" theory by George Stigler, advertising is a substitute for consumer search.[58] Advertising is an important informational device for consumers whose time is relatively valuable and/or whose efficiency in searching for a preferred provider is relatively low. Individuals with high cost of search and patient groups such as the elderly or those with limited physical capacity will perceive advertising as an effective substitute for search. Ultimately, advertising might be expected not only to substitute for a person's own search, but to increase the efficiency of the search. Extending Stigler's theory on the economics of information, we can foresee that consumers will use dental advertising to search for service characterized by —

- High absolute price (affording large savings per unit purchased)
- High dispersion of full price (money price plus time costs) among providers in a local market area
- Demand dominated by consumer groups with relatively limited access to other means of searching for low prices, high quality, and greater convenience
- High price-elasticity of demand, i.e., services for which consumer demand is sensitive to differences in price
- Infrequent purchase by the individual consumer (e.g., dentures and extractions), where the experience that comes from repetitive purchases is lacking
- Incomplete coverage by dental prepayment, so that the consumer's share of the savings from choosing a lower-priced dental care provider is significant.

Alternative theories of the economic effects of advertising focus on its role in shaping consumer tastes, but the implications are not pursued here.

Some demand-side effects of dentist advertising will influence market competition through the feedback effects between demand and supply. When advertising improves consumer awareness of alternative providers, it will lead eventually to a rise in the cross-elasticity of demand among dental practitioners. Cross-elasticity of demand measures the increase in the demand for the individual dental practice's services when the price charged by a competing practice is increased. A rise in the cross-elasticity of demand among providers enhances market competition: the difficulty of searching for low-priced dentistry contributes to local market power for individual dentists; advertising-induced reductions in consumer search costs diminish that source of market power. Improvements in the efficiency of the consumer search thus help lower dental fees.

Therefore, the principal effects of advertising on dental care costs will operate through increased competition among providers; growth of franchised and retail-based dental practices, and large dental firms; and changes in the mix of dental services as advertising-induced competition alters relative price. The six attributes of advertising discussed above suggest that some improvements in allocative efficiency will result from the informational value of advertising. In addition, increased market competition will encourage greater technical efficiency within existing practices. Finally, advertising is likely to speed the evolution of the market toward larger, low-cost dental firms.

The impact of advertising on consumer-search costs depends on the alternative informational mechanism now in use among dental care consumers. For primary dental-care services (e.g., routine oral exams, restorative and maintenance care), for example, the advice of friends, coworkers, and relatives is probably the principal source of information about prices and quality. Satterthwaite[59] discusses the importance of these sources. One might add a hypothesis to the six characteristics of advertising based on the earlier discussion of Stigler's search theory: in large markets such as urban areas, where the number of competing providers per consumer is greater, the information value of advertising (relative to informal sources in one's social network) will be higher and thus the intensity of dentist advertising will be greater. Available data showing the concentration of dental advertising in urban markets support this hypothesis.[60]

Legal restraints on claims of superiority are not likely to present significant barriers to advertising-induced price competition. This is because there is a wide range of nonliteral ways of signaling "superior" quality, not the least important of which is the apparent expense of the advertising itself. An advertisement in *Time* magazine means more than the words themselves convey. A dental practice's investment in advertising itself implies to consumers that the firm has incurred a cost that can only be recouped by increased demand for the firm's services or increased prices for those services.

The cost of advertising introduces a wedge between fees and production costs. Unless the advertisement signals some firm-specific advantage for which consumers are willing to pay a price premium, other dental practices will either mimic the firm's advertising (as in the case of advertising serving mainly to increase consumers' general awareness of dental care) or compete for the advertising firm's clients by underpricing the firm.

According to this theory, competitive market forces will discipline the dentist who advertises. The rate at which the market adjustments will occur is, of course, an empirical question. One must observe the actual workings of local dental markets over the next few years before making any definitive judgments about the efficacy of dental advertising as an indirect signal of quality and the firm's other advantages relative to other providers.

Other regulatory constraints on the time, place and manner of dental advertising will bear heavily on its ultimate competitive effect. Any entrepreneur will seek to minimize the cost of advertising messages while maximizing their impact on consumers. It is impossible a priori to sort out the potential effectiveness of radio and television advertising versus print forms of advertising. One can imagine, however, that because consumer characteristics and program preferences are correlated to some degree, the electronic media would tend to be more cost-effective in providing information about dental services.[61]

We have emphasized price advertising so far. However, "threshold" advertising—of location, office hours, and nature of practice—is a necessary precondition to the provision of price and quality information. For "experience goods" like dental services, advertising will deliver indirect information.[62] Although consumers will tend to discount advertised claims of superiority and other features of dental services that are difficult for them to evaluate, they will respond to dental advertising of location, office hours, and nature of specialty services. Even an advertisement that seems to provide little information about a particular dentist's services conveys an important signal to consumers. Because suppliers with a relative advantage in price, quality and other attributes are the ones most likely to advertise, frequency of advertising becomes an indicator of the firm's relative advantage.[63] The firm that dupes (by advertising) a substantial number of consumers will suffer a loss to its reputation proportionate to the number of persons deceived. Word-of-mouth communication among prospective patients keeps providers honest in such cases.

Evidence from two other health care markets is consistent with this procompetition model of advertising effects. Feldman and Begun's work in optometry[64] and Cady's empirical analysis of prescription drugs[65] both showed that legal restraints on advertising were related to higher prices. Empirical tests of whether the effects of advertising in dental care are consistent with other economic models—for example, the theory that advertising's major effect will be to shape consumer preferences and strengthen the loyalty of consumers to established dental providers—would represent important new knowledge for policymakers.

Certain provisions of state dental-practice acts indirectly influence the use of advertisements. For example, limits on number of dental offices per dentist, the number of dental auxiliaries per dentist, and the functions that may be delegated to dental auxiliaries place upper bounds on a dentist's capacity to expand market share. Such limits force dentists to use their own time rather than other labor inputs to increase the volume of dental services.[66] Thus, the incentive to increase patient load by advertising is dampened but not eliminated. This insight may explain why recent franchising of dental practices has been limited to practices with more than one dentist.[67] These franchise operations rely heavily on advertising—for example, the average advertising budget for the Good Care Dental Center program is estimated to be $10,000 per practice per year.

It is notable that the advertising of franchised dental practices generally does not include price information, but stresses the convenience and quality of each franchised practice. At first blush, the exclusion of price information from the advertising of dental practices whose unit costs are likely to be relatively low does not seem rational. However, the decision to focus on other attributes is consistent with an attempt by the franchised practices to market their services to as broad a consumer population as possible. Because the image of retail dentistry appears to be one of low-price, high-volume providers, such an advertising approach may allay the concerns of consumers and potential referring dentists that these practices might perform second-rate dentistry. In a market where provider-specific information on quality is limited and in which consumers may perceive a positive relationship between price and quality, advertising of low prices might be discounted heavily by consumers who place a high relative value on quality. Moreover, given that a provider's prices are considerably more flexible than technical skill[68] (which is largely determined by prior investments in human capital by the dentist and auxiliaries), the emphasis on nonprice dimensions may be the best strategy for establishing a long-term market.

Advertising of specialty services. Certain services provided by specialists, e.g., endodontics and prosthetics, offer opportunities for advertising-induced competition. Consumer information about the price of these services is relatively incomplete in ways favorable to advertising—infrequent purchase by any one consumer and a consumer-search process operating primarily through an intermediary (the referring dentist)—so dentists (especially generalists) who are new to local dental markets are likely to advertise the price of such services. Established general dentists are likely to form a second set of practitioners advertising these services. Dentists who limit their practices to a specialty area are less likely to advertise because their patients come primarily from referring dentists. The opportunity cost of advertising in terms of referral patients is probably higher for the dentist who limits his practice.

Even as dental insurance grows rapidly in the eighties, the incentive to advertise price will remain because the coinsurance rate for specialty services will be significant. In addition, the use of prior authorization[69] by dental insurance carriers requires both dentist and patient to consider price in their choice of treatment (see Chapter 6).

The extent to which advertising is used to persuade, rather than inform, dental-care consumers is a general issue in the literature on industrial organization. Some economic models posit that firms advertise services to create some monopoly power by permanently differentiating their products from those of other sellers. Without elaborating further on that position, which relies on the notion that firm-specific advertising alone can reinforce consumer loyalty to the firm's product, we wish to make clear that our analysis is derived from an alternative set of assumptions about market behavior.

An alternative explanation of the effects of persuasive advertising, which incorporates the notion that the consumer will reevaluate (and may regret) an earlier purchase decision, suggests that consumers will impose prior constraints on their purchasing behavior. T. C. Schelling has referred to this self-restraint as "the intimate contest for self-command."[70] Since consumers anticipate temptation, they try to impose constraints on themselves that will prevent regrettable decisions. Consumers who realize that dental services are purchased only infrequently offer providers the greatest opportunities for persuasive advertising. Accordingly, they are likely to discount the value of such advertisements and perhaps to rely on referrals from primary-care dentists.

One implication of our analysis is that persuasive advertising by individual dental practices is less likely to be used for primary care services such as oral prophylaxis, examinations, restorations, and periodontal care, all of which tend to be purchased repeatedly as part of an on-going dental care program. Market forces will lead to informative advertising, i.e., on price, office hours and provider characteristics, for dental services of this nature.

Conversely, persuasive advertising is potentially more effective for services such as oral surgery (e.g., extractions, maxillofacial surgery), endodontics (root canal therapy), prosthodontics, and orthodontics. However, even though these services are often done by specialists on a one-time per consumer basis and therefore seem to be plausible candidates for persuasive advertising, the professional referral network is likely to serve a quality control function for such specialty services. The cost of "regret" for these services to consumers is relatively high, but the referral structure (from primary care dentist to specialist) suggests that the costs of patient disappointment will be borne by the primary care dentist as well.

If this reasoning is correct, existing institutional arrangements and consumer/provider incentives can be expected to reduce the costs of consumer mistakes regarding quality. Nonetheless, the model of self-command pinpoints possible problem areas with respect to providers' persuasion of their patients. The consumer without a regular source of primary dental care is particularly vulnerable to persuasive claims.

The welfare costs of regret are a legitimate concern of policymakers. Measurement of the costs of mistaken choices to patients does not fall neatly into the framework of allocative and technical efficiency depicted in table 1; nevertheless they are potentially real costs. Our analysis suggests that the referral network among dentists, ongoing patient-dentist relationships, and consumer incentives will work to control (but not eliminate) such losses.

Market-expanding effects of advertising. The foregoing implications from the economics of information stand apart from any effects of advertising on the amount of demand for the service. To the extent that the absence of certain threshold information about dental providers keeps a substantial proportion of the population from seeking any dental care, however, the growth of informative advertising is likely to draw more people into the dental market. The limited empirical evidence on dentist advertising[71] seems to indicate that it does have market-expanding effects. The change in aggregate dental demand induced by advertising has not been measured, but seems to be concentrated among low-income persons and the elderly.

Early forms of dental advertising were oriented principally toward expanding the market demand for dental care. To date, the franchising concept and dental advertisements have directed their efforts at the 50 percent of the U.S. population that does not receive dental care each year.[72] Reports of dentists advertising low-cost denture services stress that many of the individuals receiving denture care from the practitioners studied had never before received professional dental care.[73] This has important implications for more general acceptance of advertising by the dental profession—promotions that increase demand for dental care are likely to be welcomed in light of the growing supply of dentists. Indeed, the ADA has conducted its own institutional advertising campaign; local dental societies have designed similar programs.[74] We hypothesize that market-expanding advertising strategies ultimately will strengthen the competitiveness of the dental care sector—the same advertising of dental-care alternatives that draws consumers into a dental practice will enhance their willingness to switch dental practices.

PREPAID DENTAL PLANS

As of December 31, 1977, 22.8 percent of the U.S. civilian population was covered by dental care prepayment plans.[75] Consumer expenditures for insured dental care has risen to 20.2 percent of dental costs since 1965, when virtually no costs (1.6 percent) were covered by prepayment. In 1982, the number of persons with dental coverage as an employment benefit is expected to reach 70 million.[76]

The trend in dental prepayment has strong implications for dental care expenditures and cost containment. Previous studies[77] have concluded that dental prepayment leads to only modest increases in the percentage of persons visiting a dentist during a year, and that the principal effect of prepayment is to redistribute expenditures toward more expensive procedures. Table 2 indicates the comparative frequency and expenditures for specific services in a large prepaid dental plan. A comparison of these data, from an insured population,

Table 2. Percentage of Patients Receiving a Service and Percentage of Total Charges for the Service in an Insured Population

Service	Percentage Receiving One or More Services/Year	Percentage of Total Charges*
Examinations	77.7	4.0
Radiographs	82.0	7.3
Prophylaxes	79.7	7.1
Amalgams and composites	64.1	25.7
Extractions	11.6	2.1
Full and partial dentures	2.5	6.7
Crowns	6.4	11.6
Bridges	3.5	18.8

Source: Data from Blue Cross and Blue Shield of Greater New York (1978).

*Approximately 17 percent of total charges are for services not included here.

with nationwide aggregate data shows that dental insurance coverage leads to significant increases in the frequency of preventive and basic restorative services (less than 50 percent of the aggregate population receive these services). This induced preventive and maintenance activity may reduce long-term dental care costs, but there is little empirical evidence on this point. A crude comparison (based on the number of decayed, missing, and filled teeth) of the 1962 U.S. population and a Blue Cross and Blue Shield subscriber group showed some evidence of better dental health in the insured group, but conclusions are limited because of the lack of an adequate control population.[78]

The most striking finding in table 2 is the skewed nature of the frequency distribution of charges: crowns and bridges were received infrequently (each by less than seven percent of the plan population), but accounted for more than 30 percent of total charges. Thus, even if the frequency of these procedures is increased slightly to reflect dental prepayment, the potential cost increases are large. Lacking empirical estimates of the price elasticity of insured dental services, qualitative remarks are the best we can offer now. For instance, the recent Rand Corporation study by Manning and Phelps[79] had little success in obtaining valid estimates of the price elasticities of crown and denture services.

Table 3. Ratio of Dental Service Demand under Full Coverage
Insurance to Demand in U.S. Population*

Age	Ratio	
0-5	4.79	
6-14	2.02	2.94
15-24	1.82	
25-44	1.46	
45-54	1.47	1.63
55+	2.32	
All Ages	1.80	

Source: Adapted from Howard L. Bailit et al., "Controlling the Cost of Dental Care," American Journal of Public Health (July 1979), pp. 699-703.
*Weighted averages for fillings, extractions, cleanings, and examinations

An earlier Rand study[80] summarized evidence from two prepaid dental plans about the effect of eliminating price on dental-care demand. Table 3 presents comparisons by age, between the utilization rate of the Group Health, Inc., of New York and the total U.S. population. The ratios suggest that the demand effects of insurance coverage are greatest for the under-25 age group, a finding confirmed in the later study by Manning and Phelps. Combining the findings of the two Rand studies, one can draw several conclusions about the expected impact of dental prepayment (full coverage) on dental care expenditures:

(1) On the average, per-capita expenditures will at least double, based on frequency of visits alone. Allowing for adjustments to service mix demand is likely to increase even more.

(2) By reducing the costs borne by patients at the point of service, dental coverage greatly reduces the sensitivity of demand to price.[81] Thus, dental-care coverage will shift consumer concerns in the direction of comparative provider amenities, quality, and convenience. On the supply side these insurance effects will induce a shift away from competition on price to the non-price dimensions of dental care.

(3) As growth in the breadth and depth of insurance subtly directs the competitive focus away from price, the burden of cost containment in the dental care sector will fall increasingly on the prepayment plan.

Cost containment from the standpoint of the prepayment plan involves several nuances. The plan's interest in containing health-care costs depends on the type of "cost." Subscriber premiums and the associated investment returns are sources of income to the plan, while claims paid and administrative costs constitute the plan's operating costs. The buyer, on the other hand, is purchasing risk reduction and a means of budgeting (prepaying) for dental service. In the face of uncertainty regarding future oral disease and therefore the need for dental care, the buyer selects a policy that smoothes income among different possible states of the world (e.g., periodontal disease and caries requiring extensive dental service vs. the complete absence of oral disease).

Understanding the nature of the service that a prepayment plan supplies—namely, risk reduction plus budgeting—is the key to clarifying the plan's economic interest in cost containment. The plan's profit incentive leads to efforts to minimize the cost of risk reduction. Specifically, the competitive plan will seek to define the coverage of a policy and introduce copayment features in such a way as to attract customers whose expected claims equal their premiums. Prepaid plans will monitor service utilization and fees to minimize losses owing to client expenditures that exceed premiums. Administrative costs will also be minimized by the profit-maximizing, competitive plan. Competition among plans (i.e., independent premium bidding to attract customers) is a central feature of this argument. Otherwise, colluding plans might realize some collective advantage by permitting dental fees and utilization to rise.

It is important to note that risk reduction has less value for prepaid dental plans than for hospital and medical plans. The financial risk related to unexpected dental expenditures is much less than for hospital and medical expenditures. Since meaningful cost containment by prepaid dental plans must stress the control of claim costs, the distinction between risk reduction and the budgeting of claim payment is key. The more consumers perceive the plan as merely an intermediary for budgeting dental expenses, the less they will demand that prepaid plans engage in cost-reducing strategies. The prevalence of patient cost-sharing, pretreatment review, and carefully drafted underwriting rules in the dental prepayment market suggest that consumers support cost-containment mechanisms, even though the potential cost savings appear to be greater in medicine.

As enrollment in dental prepayment plans continues to grow, consumer search is likely to focus on the premiums for given levels of coverage, rather than on provider fees per se. In essence, the unions, benefits compensation managers, and other agents become proxy buyers (and searchers) for the individual in the market for dental services. The group contract concentrates the market power of individual consumers and reduces the cost of collecting information about prices and provider behavior. Carriers respond to this concentrated negotiating strength by competing aggressively for group premium dollars. In turn, the carrier incentives are to negotiate cost effective contracts with dental providers.

One factor serves to weaken, but not eliminate, the dental-insurance plan's incentives for cost containment. Because employer premium contributions for health and dental insurance are exempt from federal income and Social Security payroll taxes, there is, in effect, a subsidy for premium contributions relative to wages. But the wages-versus-fringe-benefits decision is only one margin of choice. Even though that choice is distorted by a tax subsidy that is positively related to the employee's marginal tax rate (and thus provides a greater tax benefit to high-income employees), the consumer still gains by eliminating wasteful expenditures on dental care. The point is that, given the tax subsidy, a consumer will share those savings with the federal tax system. Private incentives are therefore diluted.

One can predict that prepaid dental plans will continue present strategies to control dental costs, although specific methods will need to be reevaluated. For example, the Usual, Customary, and Reasonable method of paying dentists represents a special case for cost effective reimbursement policy. Under this reimbursement system, each dentist files the usual fee for each service with the insurance carrier. The carrier generally accepts the filed fees if they are no higher than the 90th percentile of fees for dentists in the same geographic area. There is some evidence from the California Medicare and Medicaid experience that Usual, Customary, and Reasonable payments to physicians tend over time to establish a floor, rather than a ceiling, for physician fees. Holahan et al. concluded that increases in Medicare and Medicaid reasonable charges are likely to stimulate increases in physicians' actual charges to the program.[82] Their work also suggests that, if next year's reasonable charge depends on this year's actual charge, there will be a built-in inflationary bias.

An analogous study of the impact of Usual, Customary and Reasonable reimbursement in dentistry has not been done — the similarity in formulas between Medicare/Medicaid and the Usual, Customary, and Reasonable payment system in dentistry suggests that the potential price-increasing effect of Usual, Customary, and Reasonable payment ought to be examined empirically.

To put this issue into context, it should be noted that the rate of increase in dentists' fees has been relatively small (5.5 percent) from 1971 to 1975.[83] Therefore, it seems unlikely that the Usual, Customary, and Reasonable system is leading to significant inflation in dental prices. However, Usual, Customary, and Reasonable reimbursement might contribute to an increase in the fees above those that would prevail if fee schedules were of the fixed allowance or indemnity type. In addition, the growth of prepayment in the future will make Usual, Customary, and Reasonable reimbursement a more powerful market force. If Usual, Customary, and Reasonable does weaken the incentive for cost containment, then its growth via prepayment may contribute to inflation of dental fees.

In light of the preceding analysis of the incentives of prepaid dental plans, we postulate that professional "control" of third-party payers *does not* contribute significantly to the market power of dentists. Therefore, dental society sponsorship of a plan would not, by itself, lead to increased prices, reduced output, or reduced incentives to contain costs. Even if plans were to possess some market power (due to cooperation with one another), individual firms could still gain a competitive edge by monitoring and restraining providers' prices and discretionary behavior, thus lowering their premiums. Any collusion of prepaid dental plans would be especially subject to this kind of premium-cutting behavior, since the number of plans is so large as to make undetected collusion virtually impossible.

One particular court case, *Manasen v. California Dental Services* (CDS), demonstrated that dental plans act according to these incentives.

In that case, 11 practitioners challenged the dental service corporation's practice of paying substantially reduced fees to dentists who had not signed participating agreements with CDS. These agreements involved the dentist's acceptance of a ceiling for dental fees, and appear to represent a reasonable cost-containing strategy for insurers — the kind of response one would expect in a competitive prepayment market.

As the dental prepayment market grows, more competition among firms can be expected. For example, during the period 1970-76, dental service corporations' share of total dental benefit expenditures fell from 22.5 percent, to 17.7 percent. During the same interval, the share of the commercial insurers rose from 61.2 percent to 67.0 percent.[84] The rate of new entry (and the resulting competitive pressure) to the dental prepayment market is illustrated by the fact that, of 5,501 prepaid dental plans operating in 1973, 25 percent had just been established that year. Thus, market forces are likely to reinforce carriers' incentives to minimize claims and administrative costs. There is no evidence to suggest that these incentives are weaker for the dental service corporation, as compared to commercial companies and the Blue Cross and Blue Shield plans.

RECOMMENDATIONS

This chapter has explored the implications of changing supply, demand, and competitive conditions for dental-care costs in the eighties. Using the criteria of allocative and technical efficiency, the analysis suggests that competitive market forces offer a promising route to future cost containment in dentistry. A variety of natural experiments are under way in the marketplace — independent contracting for dental hygiene services, the use of satellite offices by dentists, varying degrees of delegation of expanded functions to auxiliaries, alternative forms of group practice, advertising, franchised practices, prepaid dental plans, and private insurance-claims review.

These options should be tested for economic and social viability. Specifically, state dental-practice act provisions should be reexamined in terms of their impact on dental-care costs and public health. Limits on number of offices per dentist, number of auxiliaries per dentist, and ownership of dental practices may contribute to higher dental care costs without commensurate benefits to the health of the population or in the quality of dental care.

The weakening of ethical restraints on dental advertising and other nontraditional forms of attracting patients will aid in cost containment, and offers the additional benefit of lowering the costs of reaching underserved population groups. The movement to remove collective restraints on market alternatives, whether in the form of ethical codes or legal statutes, is consistent with a subtle society-wide shift in favor of private incentives as opposed to command-and-control mechanisms for allocating resources. This trend seems likely to continue, opening the way for a fair market test of the cost-containment prospects of alternative models of dental-care delivery and financing.

Notes

1. American Dental Association, Bureau of Public Information, Public information release (Chicago, April 29, 1979).

2. Council of State Governments, *State Regulatory Policies: Dentistry and the Health Professions* (Lexington, 1979).

3. Health Resources Administration, *Forecasts of Employment in the Dental Sector to 1995* (Washington, Public Health Service, 1979).

4. The HRA projection assumes, as seems reasonable, that the rate of return to those entering the dental profession will remain sufficiently high to attract an excess of applicants relative to dental school capacity, so that the output of graduates will be determined by dental school capacity. Even so, it should be noted that the ratio of applicants to enrollment capacity is declining.

5. Robert W. Merry, "Amid the Gnashing of Teeth, Dentists Start to Advertise," *Wall Street Journal* (December 1977).

6. "Survey Results of Dentists' Income and Overhead," *Dental Economics* (May 1980), 54-58.

7. American Dental Association, *1977 Survey of Dental Practice* (Chicago, 1978).

8. Profitability is measured as the median net income of dental practices in each category (number of operatories, auxiliaries). The data show consistently increasing mean net incomes for dentists practicing alone with increases in the number of auxiliaries employed per practice.

9. Kent Nash, "Economies of Scale and Productivity of Dental Practices," paper presented at Annual Meeting of American Association for Dental Research (New Orleans, 1980).

10. Ronald Alsop, "Dental Hygienist Picks Fight with State over Right to set up Independent Practice," *Wall Street Journal* (December 30, 1980).

11. Robert A. Hankin, "The Cost of Providing Restorative Dentistry in an Alternative Delivery Mode," *Journal of Public Health Dentistry* 37(3) (1977), 217-223.

12. John Kushman, Richard Scheffler, Larry Miners, and Curt Mueller, "Non-Solo Dental Practice: Incentives and Returns to Size," *Journal of Economics and Business* (Fall 1978), 36-38.

13. Nash, "Economies of Scale."

14. Kushman et al., "Non-Solo Dental Practice."

15. Chester W. Douglass and John M. Day, "Cost and Payment of Dental Services in the United States," *Journal of Dental Education* 43(7) (1979), 330-348.

16. Kushman, et al., "Non-Solo Dental Practice."

17. American Dental Association, *American Dental Directory* (Chicago, 1970, 1976).

18. Lawrence Shepard, "Licensing Restrictions and the Cost of Dental Care," *Journal of Law and Economics* 21 (April 1978), 187-201.

19. Donald R. House, "Regulation in the Market for Dental Care: Implications for a Full Price Market-Clearing Mechanism," paper presented at annual meeting of Eastern Economic Association (Boston, May 1979).

20. For empirical estimates of dental-care demand elasticities, see Alex Maurizi, *Public Policy and the Dental Care Market* (Washington, American Enterprise Institute, 1975) and Raul Feldstein, *Financing Dental Care: An Economic Analysis* (Lexington, Lexington Books, 1973).

21. Shepard, "Licensing Restrictions."

22. *Ibid.* and House, "Regulation in the Market."

23. Douglas A. Conrad and George G. Sheldon, "Effects of Legal Constraints on Dental Care Prices," *Essays in Health Economics* (forthcoming).

24. Preston A. Littleton, Jr., "Differences between the Medical and Dental Health Care Sectors," *Journal of Dental Education*, 43 (Feburary 1979), 101-106.

25. Stanley Budner and Harriet Goldman, *Study of the Impact of Regional Boards on the Distribution of Dentists* (Washington, Department of Health and Human Services, DHPA Report No. 80-52, June 1980).

26. Betty Lee Kuhn, "A Satellite Office: Is It for You?" *Dental Management* (June 1980), 19-26.

27. Conrad, "Effects of Legal Constraints."

28. Kuhn, "A Satellite Office."

29. Council of State Governments, *State Regulatory Policies*.

30. Conrad, "Effects of Legal Constraints."

31. *The Advertising Dentist*, 1(6) (June 1980), 22-24.

32. "Drug Store Dentists," *Medical Care Review* (October 1979), 945.

33. *The Advertising Dentist*, 1(5) (May 1980), 19.

34. Donald R. House, *The Economic Relationship between Dentists' Income and Time Supplied: Final Report* (Washington, DHEW, Contract No. HRA 231-77-0177, 1978).

35. T. R. Saving, et al., *Labor Substitution and the Economics of the Delivery of Dental Services: Final Report.* (Washington, DHEW, Contract No. HRA 231-77-0135, 1978).

36. Alsop, "Dental Hygienist Picks Fight."

37. Frank A. Sloan and Roger Feldman, "Competition among Physicians," *Competition in the Health Care Sector: Past, Present, and Future*, ed. Warren Greenberg (Washington, Federal Trade Commission, 1978), 57-131.

38. Shepard, "Licensing Restrictions."

39. Donald R. House, "Dentists' Incomes, Fees, Practice Costs, and the Economic Stabilization Act: 1952 to 1976," *Journal of the American Dental Association*, 99 (November 1979), 857-861.

40. John Kushman, "Pricing Dental Services: A Market-Testing Approach," *Journal of Health Politics, Policy, and Law* (forthcoming); and Bryan Leslie Boulier, *Two Essays in the Economics of Dentistry: A Production Function for Dental Services and an Examination of the Effects of Licensure* (Ph.D. thesis, Princeton University, 1974).

41. Gerald L. Musgrave, "A Market Model of the Distribution of Dentists," *The Target Income Hypothesis and Related Issues in Health Manpower Policy* (Washington, Division of Dentistry, DHEW Publication No. HRA 80-27, 1980), 60-82.

42. Unfortunately, the HIAA data relate only to insured patients, not to the total population in the market areas in Musgrave's study. He includes proxies for the breadth of insurance coverage to correct for this problem, but it is not clear how successful such adjustments are.

43. For instance, including dentist density in the demand equation caused the price coefficient to become positive (clearly inconsistent with the law of demand) and the income elasticity to decline substantially.

44. Musgrave, "A Market Model."

45. Data on utilization and price for the noninsured population were not available. Also, estimates of the elasticity of supply with respect to price became unreasonably large in the specification he used in testing for supply-induced demand.

46. Willard G. Manning and Charles E. Phelps, *Dental Care Demand: Point Estimates and Implications for National Health Insurance* (Santa Monica, Rand Corporation, 1978).

47. Donald R. House, "A Full-Price Approach to the Dental Market: Implications for Price Determination," *Journal of Health Politics, Policy, and Law* (forthcoming).

48. Manning, *Dental Care Demand.*

49. House, "Dentists' Income."

50. The R^2 (proportion of variance in dentists' net incomes explained) of the equation was .96, but one should be cautious of the point estimates since House's scatter diagram (figure 3, p. 859) shows considerable dispersion around the predicted trend line.

51. Bureau of Economic Research and Statistics and Bureau of Public Information, Dentists' Fees and Inflation," *Journal of the American Dental Association*, 93 (July 1976), 129-133.

52. For example, it can be shown that (where ΔP_e, ΔMC represent changes in equilibrium price and in marginal cost, and E_s, E_d are absolute values of the elasticity of supply and demand, respectively)

$$\Delta P_e = \frac{\Delta MC \times E_s}{E_s + E_d}$$

53. "*Bates v. State Bar of Arizona,*" *Supreme Court Reporter*, 93 (1977), 2691.

54. American Dental Association, *Guidelines for State Boards of Dental Examiners on the Definition of Routine Dental Services for Purposes of Dentists' Advertisements* (Chicago, 1977).

55. Missouri Dental Board, *Chapter 332, RS Mo. 1969 and Rules and Regulations* (August 1978), 30-32.

56. The Rules: (1) prohibit promises of cure, relief, or improved dental health; claims of superiority over any other practitioner or reference to quality of care provided; or any announcement or advertisement by means of electronic media, e.g., radio or television; (2) permit advertising of fees *only* for routine services, following exactly the *ADA Guidelines* definition of "routine services;" and (3) specify that fee information must be definite and must include disclosures of any possible complications of post-care costs to patients.

57. American Association, Bureau of Public Information, public information release (April 29, 1979).

58. George S. Stigler, "Economics of Information," *Journal of Political Economy*, 49(3) (June 1961), 213-225.

59. Mark A. Satterthwaite, "Consumer Information, Equilibrium Industry Price, and the Number of Sellers," *Bell Journal of Economics*, 10(2) (Autumn 1979), 483-502.

60. *The Advertising Dentist* 1(5), May 1980; 1(6), June 1980.

61. For example, in a rural area the morning agricultural extension service program could be accompanied by dentist advertising. Or a special program for elderly citizens might be preceded by an advertisement of a dental practice for denture services. Both these ads would reach customarily low-use customers.

62. Nelson classifies characteristics of economic commodities into two broad groups: experience qualities and search characteristics. The former can be ascertained only by the consumer using the good, while the latter can be judged by searching among alternative suppliers without actually purchasing the good. Quality is predominantly an experience characteristic, while such factors as price are search characteristics.

63. This argument depends on long-term learning by consumers. Intensive advertising will draw consumers in the short run to the firm doing the advertising; but, if the firm has no real advantage over other suppliers (who also advertise), consumers will ultimately drift to other firms until market shares reflect comparative performance.

64. Roger Feldman and James Begun, "Effects of Advertising: Lessons from Optometry," *Journal of Human Resources*, XIII (special supplement) (1978), 247-262.

65. John Cady, *Restricted Advertising and Competition: The Case of Retail Drugs* (Washington, American Enterprise Institute, 1976).

66. T. R. Saving, *et al.*, *Labor Substitution and the Economics of the Delivery of Dental Services* (Washington, DHEW, Contract No. HRA-231-77-0135, 1978).

67. Chris Corby, "The Birth of Franchise Dentistry," *Dental Economics* (May 1979), 53-55.

68. A similar argument applies to convenience of location and the modernity of the practice's dental equipment and technology, both of which represent investments in capital that are fixed in the short run.

69. This is the procedure by which proposed treatment plans are submitted by the dentist to the carrier for review and approval by a dental consultant. Ordinarily, only treatment plans whose total price would exceed, say $100 to $150, are subject to prior authorization.

70. T. C. Schelling, "The Intimate Contest for Self-Command," *The Public Interest* (Summer 1980).

71. The Advertising Dentist, 1(5) May 1980; Irvin Molotsky, "Dentists, Other Professionals Finding It Pays to Advertise," *New York Times* (January 17, 1978).

72. Corby, "The Birth of Franchise Dentistry."

73. Molotsky, "Dentists, Other Professionals."

74. American Dental Association, "Pilot Institutional Ad Campaign Resumes," *ADA News* (August 18, 1980), 1.

75. Carroll, "Private Health Insurance."

76. Howard L. Bailit, Melvin Raskin, Susan Reisine, and Douglas Chiriboga, "Controlling the Cost of Dental Care," *American Journal of Public Health*, 69(7) (July 1979), 699-703.

77. ADA, "Pilot Institutional Ad Campaign"; Bailit, et al., "Controlling the Cost of Dental Care."

78. Howard L. Bailit and Melvin Raskin, "Assessing Quality of Care and Dental Insurance," *Inquiry*, 15(4) (December 1978), 358-370.

79. Manning and Phelps, *Dental Care Demand*.

80. Lorraine A. Clasquin, *Mental Health, Dental Services, and Other Coverage in the Health Insurance Study* (Santa Monica: Rand Corporation, R-1216-OEO, November 1973).

81. For example, the estimates of Manning and Phelps suggest that the price elasticity of dental care demand for white children drops (in absolute value) from -1.40 to -0.26 in going from full market prices to dental care at 25 percent of market price.

82. John Holahan, et al., *Physician Pricing in California: Final Report* (Washington, DHEW, Contract No. 600-76-0054, 1978).

83. Bureau of Economic Research, "Dentists' Fees and Inflation."

84. Marjorie Smith Carroll and H. Arnett Ross, III, "Private Health Insurance Plans in 1977: Coverage, Enrollment, and Financial Experience," *Health Care Financing Review*, 1(2) (Fall 1979), 3-22.

2

The Delivery of Dental Care

Howard L. Bailit and Robert T. Kudrle

INTRODUCTION

Until recently the system for delivering personal dental services in the United States remained relatively unchanged with most care provided by solo dentists in fee-for-service practice who received direct payment from patients after completion of treatment. Although the traditional delivery system still predominates, substantial changes are now taking place relating to prepayment for services, group practices, capitation payment methods, relocation of traditional practice sites, regulation of professional behavior, and new technologies. This chapter will examine how these changes may affect the cost of dental care.

Here we introduce a conceptual framework that considers dental providers and payers as sharing in the ultimate decisions concerning allocation of treatment resources: providers decide on the care needed and payers determine demand. These decisions lead to expenditures for the facilities, equipment, supplies, and manpower required to deliver services.

As seen in figure 1, the decisions of providers and payers are influenced by complex interactions among the major components of the delivery system. For example, although a dentist's decision to

The authors are grateful to Douglas Conrad, John Kushman, and Max Schoen for their detailed critical comments on earlier versions of this chapter. They bear no responsibility, however, for the errors of evidence, logic, or wisdom that remain.

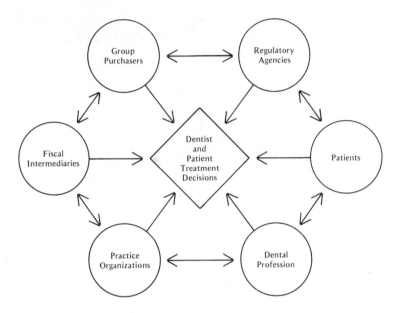

Figure 1. Interactions Among Major Components of the Dental Care Delivery System

provide a particular set of services is determined mainly by the dental health of the patient, other considerations also come into play. These include the patient's ability to pay for recommended services, the dentist's financial incentives associated with a particular payment method, resource constraints of the dental practice, and structural or process-level regulatory controls imposed by public or private agencies.

If dentists have incentives to behave in certain ways, so do the different types of payers; patients, fiscal intermediaries, and group purchasers of dental care. These incentives are derived from each group's objectives in the dental delivery system. Although the objectives of each group are varied, table 1 presents what may be considered their primary objectives.

Because this is a complex topic, the chapter starts with a more detailed specification of the issues and with an examination of the assumptions made in developing major themes. The next section reviews delivery-system incentives on provider behaviors and considers the influence of practice organization and payment methods. The chapter then turns to payer incentives and explores the effects of dental-benefit plans, regulatory systems, industrial and school-based dental clinics, and patient decisions on the cost of care. We conclude with a general discussion.

Table 1. Primary Objectives of Major Groups in Dental Care Delivery Systems

Interest Group	Primary Incentives
Patients	Maximize (perceived) well-being by:* ° seeking to reduce full price of dental services ° seeking to increase health-effectiveness of dental services
Group Purchasers	Maximize profits or (for nonprofit organizations) ensure solvency and growth by: ° lowering total expenditures ° maintaining or increasing beneficiary satisfaction
Fiscal Intermediaries	Maximize profits or (for non-profit organizations) assume solvency and growth by: ° minimizing costs while maintaining adequate dentist participation ° setting premium prices as high in relation to costs as competition will allow ° maintaining or increasing beneficiary satisfaction
Dental Profession	Increase net professional incomes for a standard work week Enhance the status of the profession Improve the dental health of the community

*Instrumental objectives to be combined or traded off against each other

SPECIFICATIONS AND ASSUMPTIONS

Before examining the effect of delivery system components on provider and payer incentives, five basic issues need further discussion.

1. The term "dental delivery system" is used here to include the multiple and varied methods for providing personal dental services to the American people. Thus, there is no one delivery system but rather many different systems and subsystems that are often in competition.
2. Throughout the chapter reference is made to delivery-system changes that might improve dental health. These improvements are considered broadly to include outcomes such as reduction in pain and disability, prevention and cure of caries and periodontal disease, and improved social functioning. It is clear that dental health is a multi-dimensional concept that is not easily defined. Also, the relationship between dental health and the delivery system is complex. However, this chapter assumes that, at the aggregate level, provision of more dental services leads to improvement in dental health.
3. The cost of dental care is directly related to the efficiency of the dental-care delivery system. Efficiency is defined in three principal ways: (1) minimizing the cost of producing a unit of

service of standard quality; (2) minimizing the cost of producing a unit of dental health; and (3) minimizing the difference between the cost of producing an additional unit of service and the purchase price of the additional service. The third definition is considered in Chapter 1 and will not be pursued further.

It is important to clarify the difference between the first two definitions. The cost of producing an amalgam restoration, for example, could remain constant, but if a new amalgam material were used that prevented subsequent decay, dental health would increase, since the restoration presumably would last longer. Thus, the cost of producing health would decrease, but the dollar cost of restoring the tooth would remain the same. The result would be a more efficient delivery system.

4. It is also important to stress that this chapter does not make any assumptions about reducing total expenditures for dental care. There could be substantial improvements in delivery-system efficiencies and at the same time large increases in total expenditures. This could occur if more people received more and better quality care. A strong case can be made that unlike medicine, increased use of basic dental services by the American people would lead to significant increases in dental health as total dental expenditures climbed.

5. The final assumption that needs to be made explicit relates to expected delivery-system changes during the next ten years. The position taken in this chapter is that changes will occur incrementally and that major restructuring is unlikely. Therefore, the chapter focuses on present trends in the delivery of dental care rather than on possible radical changes in the system.

With these background definitions and assumptions, we turn to the influences of the delivery system on provider behavior, starting with the impact of dental-practice organizations.

PROVIDER INCENTIVES AND THE COST OF CARE

The major organizational factors related to practice-production efficiency are the number of dentists per practice, ownership of practice, and payment methods. Because of their importance and complexity, payment methods are considered separately.

Current Trends in Organizations

It is estimated that 95 percent of dental services are provided in the offices of 103,000 dentists who own or are employed in private practices.[1] Of these, 71 percent were in solo practice in 1977. There were increasing numbers of two-dentist offices, where dentists in the same facility either share expenses but not profits or share both expenses and profits; approximately 14 percent of dentists practiced with one other dentist.[2] Group practices, defined as three or more dentists who share expenses and profits, are also increasing but still include only 8 percent of practices. The great majority of group practices have three to five dentists (a small percentage have 10 or more dentists) and are made up of general dentists. Few group practices include both generalists and specialists or a mix of specialists.[3]

Private dental firms are almost always owned by at least one of the dentists providing care in the practices. Offices where one dentist employs other dentists are becoming more common as department store-based and large advertising practices become established in urban centers.[4]

Another growing form of private practice is industry-owned and -operated dental clinics. Few now exist, but they are attracting more attention as companies attempt to control employee health care costs.[5]

The method of paying for dental services is predominantly fee-for-service. Less than 1 percent of practices are prepaid groups or Independent Practice Associations (IPAs) receiving capitation payments.[6] One recent development is insurance-carrier-operated networks of affiliated, dentist-owned solo or group practices.[7] Patients are given the choice of receiving care in affiliated practices with reduced out-of-pocket expenses or in nonaffiliated practices. Carriers reimburse affiliated practices under a capitation plan in which practices assume most of the financial risk.

In addition to privately owned practices approximately 1,600 hospitals (about 30 percent) have dental clinics that offer outpatient care.[8]

Finally, there are publicly owned and operated nonhospital dental clinics that provide care to groups of special concern to the public, such as armed forces personnel, prisoners, American Indians, institutionalized retarded children, veterans and, recently, the medically indigent. It is estimated that about 5 million people are eligible for care in the public system.[9] These are usually group practices employing salaried civilian or military dentists.

Organization and Efficiency

Dental-practice surveys report that group practitioners have 20 to 30 percent higher incomes than solo dentists.[10] The obvious question is whether these higher incomes reflect greater efficiency in group practices. For most goods and services, there are economies of scale — larger production units are more efficient. Theoretically, this could obtain in dentistry, where group practices, and especially large group practices, could produce services at a lower unit cost than solo or small group practices. Possible reasons for such a relationship are given in table 2.

Table 2. Theoretical Advantages of Group Practices in Reducing the Unit Cost of Producing Services Through Economies of Scale

	Division of labor allowing dentists and other personnel to specialize and thereby become more proficient
Labor Factors	Better use of auxiliary personnel
	Availability of colleagues for diagnostic consultation and referral
	Professional management
Technological Factors	Ability to purchase and utilize more efficient and/or advanced equipment
	More efficient use of facilities (i.e., extended office hours)
Financial Factors	Discounts on large orders of materials
	Decreasing interest rates with increasing loan size

The evidence is limited but a few reports are available. Douglass and Nash[11] did not find any significant difference in the number of patient visits per dentist-hour with increasing practice size. When they used gross billings generated per dentist-hour (another productivity measure), the researchers found that two- and three-dentist practices were more productive than solo practices but no less productive than larger group practices. They noted, however, that these findings might have resulted from different service mixes among practices, and from the fact that gross billings do not differentiate between dental-production costs and fees.

In contrast, Kushman et al.,[12] and Kushman and Nuckton[13] found substantial profitability with increasing size in nonsolo dental practices. These results are interesting but must be considered tentative, because the production functions used in the estimates calculated visitation rates by combining patients of dentists and hygienists and did not control for service mix.

Some indirect evidence on economies of scale comes from the previously noted trend toward increased practice size. This trend might be viewed as evidence from "survivor analysis" that larger practices are more efficient. Kushman[14] also reported that nonsolo practices tend to accept more Medicaid patients, who pay lower fees. He speculated that nonsolo practices may find Medicaid patients more attractive because of lower production costs.

Our conclusion from the review of the literature is that there may well be economies of scale beyond the solo or two-dentist pratice. Yet, available studies are so limited that any numerical estimates of such economies should be used with extreme caution. Investigations of nonhospital medical practices suggest that whatever the extent of such economies, they may be lost in group practices of moderate size.[15]

It has also been suggested that group practices are more efficient in producing dental health because they provide superior quality care.[16] Three main reasons for this are hypothesized. First, dentists in groups may tend to concentrate on certain procedures and become adept at providing them. Second, formal and informal peer systems may operate in larger organizations. In a large group of dentists and auxiliaries, explicit rules and regulations are needed in areas such as uniform patient record systems or formal review procedures for patient complaints. Finally, even without formal systems, dentists in group practice have the opportunity to see each others' patients and evaluate each other's work. To maintain the respect of professional peers, each dentist has an incentive to perform at a level acceptable to the group.

The evidence to support these hypotheses is not available. Furthermore, even if the quality of care is superior in group practice, it is not known if the dental health of patients is better, or if better, whether it is produced at lower costs.

However, a number of studies have compared the quality of care in solo and group medical practices, both fee-for-service and prepaid.[17] The data suggest that, in general, group practices do provide better care. However, the groups studied are usually associated with medical schools, large hospitals or other nonprofit associations. These types of group practices may not be representative; the examination of a random selection of groups might show different results.

Ownership

Several issues are of concern relating to ownership. In most states only dentists can legally own practices or employ dentists to provide care.[18] The ostensible reason for this restriction is the assumption that nondentists would tend to reduce the quality of patient care in an effort to maximize profits. Conversely, it is assumed that dentists, although interested in profits, are trained to respect professional ethics that give priority to patient welfare. Data to support or reject this argument are not available, but questions can be raised about its validity.

Profit-motivated private industry in the United States responsibly produces many goods and services that have a greater impact on health and general welfare than dental care. There is good reason to believe that, on average, industry would act with equal responsibility in operating dental offices. Although some quality-assurance monitoring would be necessary, this is also true of dentist-owned practices. Therefore, questions of quality are not very compelling in arguments about nondentist ownership of dental practices.

Of greater relevance is the effect of nondentist ownership on the cost of dental care. One possibility is that allowing nondentist ownership would attract capital that could be used to create larger and better equipped, staffed and managed dental practices. While little data are available to support this position, there are reasons to doubt that current ownership restrictions are of critical importance in capital formation. The main one is that many dentists already are able to raise sufficient private capital to create large-scale practices.[19] This does not mean, of course, that large, established corporations could not generate more capital than a group of dentist entrepreneurs.

However much capital is needed, it is evident that major investments by dentists or nondentists in large dental networks are uncommon. This suggests that the presumed economic advantage of large-scale dental practices may not be sufficient to attract entrepreneurs. Furthermore, no one has demonstrated that more capital, facilities, equipment, or nondentist professional management would significantly increase dental-practice efficiency.

Another suggested advantage of nondentist ownership is an increased willingness to try new business and patient-care methods that, until recently, were considered unethical by the dental profession. Examples include advertising, capitation payment plans, and use of expanded-duty auxiliaries. Although most of these practices are now considered ethical, there is still peer pressure among dentists to maintain traditional values. Nondentists presumably would not be subject to the pressure of tradition and might be more willing to experiment with new organizational forms. However, significant numbers of dentists presumably are not affected by peer pressure and have the same incentives to innovate as nondentists. The increasing number of dentists who advertise and operate "discount" practices supports this conclusion.

It appears, then, that nondentist ownership of dental practices may have little effect on production efficiency. This, of course, does not imply that present ownership restrictions are in the public interest. It does suggest that nondentist ownership would not by itself lead to a major restructuring of the dental-care system.[20]

Hospital-owned ambulatory dental clinics. Many nonprofit hospitals have outpatient dental departments that offer general dental or oral surgical care. Such clinics range in size from one- to multi-chair facilities, but most have three or fewer chairs. The efficiency of these clinics has not been studied extensively, but some data suggest that their operating expenses exceed most privately owned dental practices.[21] The reason for this probably relates to such factors as employment of part-time salaried or volunteer dentists, support of dental-resident education programs, high broken-appointment rates, dependence on hospital support systems, and insufficient working capital. It is unlikely that the cost of producing dental services in these clinics could be reduced to approach that in private practices.

Publicly owned dental clinics. Federal, state, and local governments operate dental clinics for special populations that do not receive care in the private sector. These dental facilities represent a broad range of different organizational types, manpower configurations, practice sizes, and locations. Therefore, it is difficult to generalize about their efficiency. There is increasing evidence that salaried dentists have lower productivity[22] and the conventional wisdom is that dentists working under civil-service or military work rules do not work as efficiently as self-employed dentists. Data on per-visit costs in Neighborhood Health Centers seem to support the latter position.[23]

In contrast, Swedish evidence suggests similar productivity for publicly employed and private dentists,[24] and studies of programs for children in North America have found either comparable productivity or even an advantage in productivity for public dental personnel.[25]

As a tentative conclusion, public sector salaried dentists probably are less efficient than their fee-for-service counterparts, but the evidence is far from conclusive. Furthermore, proponents of public ownership of health programs argue that efficiency studies so far have not allowed for differences in the types and severity of illness and psycho-social problems of patients served so as to permit valid comparisons.[26] Hence, even if public programs have higher costs relative to the rest of the dental-care sector, they have to be valued in terms of the social benefits provided to populations that have difficulty obtaining services in the private sector. Still others suggest that underserved populations could be served more effectively by private dentists paid by public funds.

In conclusion, the data do not conclusively confirm that practices larger than several dentists are significantly more efficient. With respect to practice ownership, nondentist practices are unlikely to lead to major gains in efficiency.

Ownership of dental practices by nonprofit voluntary groups and governments probably reduces practice efficiency compared to privately owned practices. Publicly owned practices now serve an essential function providing care to patients who have difficulty obtaining these services in the private sector, although the role of private practice here could perhaps be greater with stronger incentives.

Payment Methods and Efficiency

This section examines the impact of payment methods on the efficiency of dental-care delivery. To begin, we discuss five common characteristics of prepaid dental care and then the difference in incentives between fee-for-service and capitation payment.

With respect to prepaid dental care: (1) Dental insurance is not "insurance" in the same sense as life insurance that involves high cost and unpredictable events occurring at a known rate throughout the population. Since almost everyone has some form of treatable dental disease, dental insurance is actually a prepaid budget plan with premiums calculated on the basis of actuarial predictions of utilization by the insured group; (2) The demand for dental services is more elastic than many other health-care services: a reduction in out-of-pocket payment results in a substantial increase in the amount of service demanded; (3) The demand for dental services varies greatly across the population according to a number of patient characteristics, including education, income, and age; (4) A few expensive and often elective services (e.g., crowns and bridges) account for a large share of total dental-care expenditures and dental-insurance benefits. Because of variations in need and typically high coinsurance rates, only a small percentage of enrollees receive these services; (5) The lower prices resulting from insurance create a tendency for all insureds to consume more than they would otherwise, raising dental-insurance premiums well above what average dental expenditures would be in the absence of insurance. Also, there is the added administrative cost of the insurance itself. Taken together, these factors suggest that, in the absence of other considerations, budgeting dental expenses through dental insurance would be very expensive for the average person compared to simply paying out-of-pocket for services.

The primary reason there is so much dental insurance is that under the present federal tax law, dental insurance purchased by employers is untaxed income for employees, hence lowering the price of insurance significantly below what it would otherwise be. These comments on prepaid dental care apply to both fee-for-service and capitation payment methods.

Now, turning to the incentives of these payment systems, under fee-for-service payment dentists have financial inducements to produce services efficiently[27] and to recommend as much service as is consonant with patient needs and professional ethics.[28] Fee-for-service payment may thus be expected to lead to both high productivity and higher total expenditures. The major potential problem associated with this payment method is overtreatment.

With respect to capitation payment, a distinction needs to be made between providers that employ dentists and providers that actually deliver care. In capitation programs, owners of prepaid groups can reimburse employee dentists by different methods (e.g., straight salary, salary with a production bonus) so that employee dentists may have different financial incentives from practice owners. However, it is assumed that regardless of how employee dentists are paid, practice owners will establish utilization controls in response to the incentives of capitation payment.[29] Therefore, agreeing to provide dental care under capitation payment methods gives dental-practice owners the financial incentive to provide fewer services per patient and, where possible, to substitute less costly services. Further, since dentists under capitation payment methods are typically paid a salary, they may tend to produce fewer services per unit time, although some complex incentive payment schemes have been devised.[30] Taking both considerations together, capitation payment can be expected to lead to lower productivity and total expenditures. The major potential problem associated with this payment method is undertreatment.

Effect on efficiency. With these generalizations in mind, the effects of capitation and fee-for-service payment systems on practice efficiency and total expenditures can be examined. In terms of the cost of raising the level of dental health, capitation programs may be more efficient for several reasons. First, where enrolled populations are stable, the operators of capitation plans have the financial incentive to encourage preventive services that reduce the incidence of disease and the need for curative treatments. This, of course, assumes that it is always cheaper to prevent rather than to treat dental disease. The evidence on the cost-effectiveness of preventive services in dental practices is insufficient to establish the validity of this assumption.

A second potential advantage lies in the fact that capitation practices have a defined patient population and could, if motivated, attempt to allocate proportionately more resources to those with the poorest dental health. This strategy is not feasible in a fee-for-service system, where patients traditionally are treated on demand.

This seeming advantage of capitation payment plans may be difficult to obtain, practically. There would be substantial expense screening large numbers of patients and setting priorities for their treatment, and considerable dissatisfaction may be generated when patients are asked to wait for treatment they perceive as necessary or to obtain treatment they perceive as unnecessary. Certainly, there is abundant evidence that patient attitudes are a major determinant of utililization, even when financial barriers to dental care are removed.[31] Therefore, even though the allocation of treatment resources by patient need rather than demand is a possibility in capitation plans, there are likely to be serious problems with this approach.

It has also been postulated that capitation practices might provide better quality services because their financial incentives are to have patients reach maintenance levels of care as soon as possible. The problem with this argument is that, except for very poor care, the relationship between quality of dental service and improved dental health is not clearly established. Hence, even if the quality of care were somewhat superior in capitation practices, this does not necessarily mean that increased dental health would result.

Effect on total expenditure. In terms of total expenditures capitation systems are also thought to have an advantage because dentists are at financial risk with a fixed budget. However, an opposing argument suggests that capitation programs that reduce patient out-of-pocket costs should increase total expenditures.

On the savings side, dentists in capitation practices can control utilization by seeing patients less frequently, providing fewer services per patient, selecting less costly alternative services when possible, and attempting to prevent disease. Presumably these controls over utilization would reduce total expenditures but would not decrease dental health.

The opposing view is that capitation plans that reduce patient out-of-pocket costs will increase utilization and, therefore, total expenditures. The rationale for this position is based on the significant price elasticity of dental-service demand and on the assumption that most Americans have considerable unmet dental-care needs. Fee-for-service dentists have the incentive to provide the necessary care—and perhaps to overtreat—and are constrained mainly by their patients' inability to pay. If capitation payment plans encourage more patients to accept necessary care, the total cost may exceed any savings gained from reducing the overtreatment seen in fee-for-service practices.

Table 3. Pretreatment Review of Dental Claims Based on Radiographic Evidence.

	Approved Services	Denied Services	No Decision	Additional Services
Fillings				
Dollars	22,019	7,041	36,916	14,945
Number of services	(834)	(300)	(2006)	(815)
Percentage of total requested expenditures	33	11	56	23
Crowns				
Dollars	73,405	14,864	40,889	15,054
Number of services	(404)	(71)	(245)	(91)
Percentage of total requested expenditures	56	12	32	12
Endodontics				
Dollars	18,757	665	18,612	8,704
Number of services	(121)	(8)	(124)	(53)
Percentage of total requested expenditures	49	2	49	23
Periodontics				
Dollars	24,594	3,975	19,527	141,048
Number of services	(304)	(58)	(210)	(310)
Percentage of total requested expenditures	51	8	41	293
Partial bridges				
Dollars	30,432	775	4,144	4,202
Number of services	(121)	(6)	(40)	(16)
Percentage of total requested expenditures	86	2	12	12
Fixed bridge units (crowns and pontics)				
Dollars	139.719	18,485	45,133	5,598
Number of services	(663)	(90)	(215)	(29)
Percentage of total requested expenditures	69	9	22	3
Extractions				
Dollars	17,929	2,330	10,814	1,239
Number of services	(242)	(65)	(156)	(50)
Percentage of total requested expenditures	56	8	35	4
Total expenditures	$326,855	$48,135	$176,035	$190,790

Dental payment plans. Empirical, indirect evidence for payment-system efficiencies comes from recent studies of dental payment plans by Bailit and his colleagues.[32] They reported what trained dental examiners found from examination of patients and radiographs assessing the necessity and appropriateness of services listed on pretreatment claims. The patients were covered by a comprehensive insurance plan that paid for 80 percent of UCR charges and included a small family deductible. As seen in table 3, the cost of services added to treatment plans exceeded money saved through denials. Even insured patients with substantially reduced out-of-pocket costs still did not receive many services, especially periodontal services, that would have benefited them.

Additional evidence of restriction of services comes from a survey of utilization of treatments such as periodontal scalings and bridges compared to estimates of population dental-health status.[33] Insurance claim data from several carriers indicated that less than 10 percent of adult eligibles visiting the dentist annually received one or more periodontal scalings or bridge service. In comparison epidemiological studies suggest that well over 50 percent of adults have periodontal disease and missing teeth.

Because these findings run counter to the expected effects of fee-for-service incentives, the reasons for undertreatment by fee-for-service dentists deserves discussion. The main reason may be the reluctance of patients to commit the necessary money and time to obtain needed care. Even in the "richer" dental-insurance plans, many services have 20 to 50 percent coinsurance charges, so that patients still have substantial out-of-pocket costs.

Perhaps of equal importance, patients may be unwilling to spend long hours in the dental chair and to experience the anxiety and pain associated with many dental services. It is also likely that some dentists fail to recognize pathology or decide not to provide care because the treatment is beyond their abilities.

If interpreted correctly, these data indicate that undertreatment is widespread in the fee-for-service system. Therefore, even if overtreatment associated with fee-for-service payment were reduced by the incentives of capitation payment, the net effect might be to increase total demand as patient out-of-pocket charges are lowered.

As noted previously, data directly comparing fee-for-service and capitation dental plans are limited, and the few reports available have methodological problems. The earliest and perhaps best study was done by Schoen,[34] who compared capitation and fee-for-service patients in the same group practice. He reported few differences in the mix of services. In a later study Schoen[35] compared utilization of services in a capitation group and open-panel practices. The group practice achieved much higher utilization rates for visits, prophylaxes, and removable partial dentures. Rates for extractions, crowns, and bridges were similar.

In similar investigations by Rosen, et al.[36] and Cogan,[37] capitation patients were found to have received more preventive services and the same or fewer bridges; the remaining utilization differences did not show a clear pattern. Finally, Olsen and Chetelat[38] found that utilization of routine procedures was generally similar for patients under the two payment plans but the capitation plan provided fewer bridges and fewer complex periodontal procedures.

It is difficult to draw conclusions from these studies because there are many factors other than payment methods that could account for the results. It is not clear, for example, whether patients in the two payment groups were comparable in dental-health status, education, number of children, and other variables known to influence utilization. Furthermore, even when these variables are controlled, generalizing from experiences in only a few dental practices is obviously difficult.

Medical capitation plans. The literature on medical capitation practices is richer and has been summarized by Luft.[39] It appears that Health Maintenance Organizations obtain savings on the order of 10 to 40 percent mainly because their hospital admission rates are 30 percent or more lower than those of conventionally insured populations. Apparently, there are few other differences between fee-for-service and capitation practices in the average length of hospital stay, ambulatory visit rates, or technical efficiency in delivering ambulatory or hospital care. In other words, HMOs appear to save money principally by delivering fewer services, not through the use of alternative production methods. Because it is not clear that any major category of dental services could be cut in a way that is analogous to "excess hospitalization," there is reason to doubt that a proliferation of capitation-payment methods in dentistry could significantly reduce costs without the possibility of serious decline in quality.

In conclusion, several theoretical but not very convincing arguments suggest that practices reimbursed under a capitation-payment system should be more efficient and have lower total expenditurẹs. It is difficult to draw any conclusions because so few well-controlled studies have compared fee-for-service and capitation dental-practice systems, and the efficiencies obtained in medical capitation programs, mainly reduced hospital admissions, are not available to dental capitation plans.

PAYER INCENTIVES AND THE COST OF CARE

Three types of direct dental-care payment groups can be identified. Governments use tax revenues to fund public dental programs and employers and labor unions set up funds to purchase dental-insurance plans for workers. Fiscal intermediaries that administer the funds constitute a second group. Included here are insurance companies, self-insured trusts, and public agencies such as state-run Medicaid programs. A third group includes patients or potential patients who buy dental services for themselves or for others, either directly out-of-pocket or indirectly through fringe benefits and taxes.

As noted previously (see table 1), all three classes of payers have financial incentives to seek delivery-system economies. Patients with insurance coverage have the additional incentive to use insured care to reduce their out-of-pocket costs. Thus, for insured patients there is a conflict between individual and group incentives to control costs.

The strategies available to payers to achieve these goals obviously differ by type of payer. Group purchasers and fiscal intermediaries can (1) construct benefit packages that maximize the dental health produced for the dollars expended; (2) develop regulatory systems that attempt to control provider behavior; and (3) operate their own dental practices in the work-place or local community. These three strategies are not mutually exclusive.

Benefit Plan Structures

Dental insurance plans must specify the services covered and any restrictions on their use; the financial constraints on utilization such as deductibles and coinsurance; and the method for paying dentists under the fee-for-service system. Mainly through financial restraints on patients, insurance-plan benefit structures influence the services patients receive and, in turn, presumably their dental health. Thus benefit plans that result in patients receiving a particular set of services could have important effects on dental health resulting from given levels of expenditures. The problem is identifying the benefit structures that lead to utilization of appropriate sets of services.

Presumed relationships among benefit structures, utilization of services, and dental health are already reflected in dental insurance plans. Yet, the relationships are complex. The profit-seeking insurance company can succeed only by offering a benefit package that enhances dental health if the plan is attractive to the group purchaser and the patient. Furthermore, problems of unstable client groups and pre-existent conditions also help shape the benefit package. Most plans cover basic diagnostic, preventive, and simple restorative procedures and have low patient contributions to enhance utilization of the services. In contrast, expensive services such as crowns or bridges usually have high coinsurance charges.

Assuming that consumers do value better dental health, additional gains in efficiency are possible through modification in benefit structures. However, more information is required on the number, mix, and sequences of services that result in improved health for particular groups of patients. It is also necessary to know how much health is improved for the dollars expended. These issues are just beginning to be explored by clinical researchers. The main point is that increases in the efficiency of raising the level of dental health could be obtained if more information were available on the cost-effectiveness of certain services and patterns of care. With this information it might be possible to construct benefit plans that offer patients and dentists economic incentives toward efficiently delivered and needed services.

Regulatory Systems

Payers interested in cost-saving also can establish regulations to modify the behavior of dentists. Regulations at the structural level include relicensure requirements; at the process level they include pretreatment review systems. It is important to note that regulations can be established by public regulatory agencies (e.g., state boards of dental examiners) or by contractual agreements among purchasers, fiscal intermediaries, and dentists.

Structural regulations. Assuming that better-educated dentists are more efficient producers of dental health—a reasonable but undocumented assumption—then substantial progress already has been made in the past 75 years through structural regulations by the establishment of university-based dental-education systems that require fundamental knowledge of science. This is a far cry from the proprietary dental-school training of the early 1900s that resulted in the graduation of dental tradesmen comparable to the denturist of today.[40] These advances were brought about through dental accreditation programs, licensure laws, and similar regulations.

Whether additional progress can be made through structural-level regulations is problematic. In public regulation, there has been discussion about requiring graduate dentists to take a year of residency training before being eligible for a license. Practicing dentists also could be required to take continuing education credits or even periodic examinations for relicensure or recertification.[41] Beyond these suggestions concerning dentist knowledge and skills, there is the possibility of changing dental-practice acts to expand the duties of auxiliaries. The role of auxiliaries is further considered in Chapter 3 and will not be discussed here.

Other structural options available to payers include requiring specific educational qualifications, such as specialty board status, before declaring a dentist eligible for reimbursement for certain services. Perhaps only board-eligible or qualified prosthodontists could receive payment for complex prosthetic services. Because prosthodontists presumably have special expertise, they may provide higher quality prosthodontic services in less time, resulting in improved efficiency, but such a case remains to be made. In our view, then, it is questionable whether such regulations would significantly increase dental-practice efficiency.

Process regulations. Payer regulation of dental-care processes has taken two different forms, but both attempt to prevent overutilization of expensive services. One strategy has been to specify in the insurance contract that certain services, believed to be overused, are not covered. Thus, some carriers do not pay for double abutments in prosthetic cases. While a legitimate case can be made for double abutments in certain situations, the carriers argue that it is better to exclude the service from the benefit package and require patients needing double abutments to pay for one crown out-of-pocket. The exclusion reduces program administrative costs of reviewing each double abutment claim and, of course, the cost of the additional crown. The savings permit premiums to be lowered or allow other benefits to be added to the insurance plan. Hence, patients in aggregate may benefit from this type of regulatory control.

A further process-level control employed by insurance carriers is to limit the fees paid on insurance claims to some given percentage of filed fees. It is not known how much the insurers save through this practice and how savings affect premiums; it is likely that the savings are considerable, however. Furthermore, with an increasing dentist-population ratio, there is little chance that this control will be modified because of practitioner pressure.

Another process-level regulation requires dentists to submit claims and radiographs for cases over some specified dollar amount before treatment begins. These claims are reviewed to determine, if the patient is eligible, if the services are covered, and if the services are necessary and appropriate under the terms of the contract. Appropriateness is determined by dental consultants employed by carriers. This system, known as pretreatment review (among other names), results in the examination by dental consultants of 3 to 5 percent of claims.[42] Services denied can still be provided, but patients must pay for them out-of-pocket.

One study estimated net savings from contractual and professional denials to be 7 and 3 percent, respectively, of total premium dollars.[43] In addition, dentists know that some of their claims will be professionally reviewed, which may make them more conservative in planning treatment. This implicit effect of pretreatment review is reported to save about 10 percent of claim costs.[44]

Pretreatment review systems save money for purchasers and fiscal intermediaries, but the question of their effect on dental-practice efficiency remains. Most savings are from the contractual denial of services, i.e., the services may be necessary, but they are not covered benefits. Such denials probably do not influence efficiency; they do decrease total expenditures.

Denials as they relate to the necessity of requested services are a more complex problem. Assuming that consultant decisions are valid, the implication is that less expensive but acceptable services would lead to comparable health outcomes. In this way consultant reviews protect carriers' financial liability and at the same time may increase the efficiency of treatment plans in raising the level of dental health while saving money.

Whether dental health is improved, of course, depends on the response of dentists and patients. If patients decide to go ahead with treatment and pay for denied services, then there are no real savings but merely transfer of costs from insurance carriers to patients. Some data suggest that in only 18 percent of denials, depending on the service, do patients pay for them out-of-pocket.[45] Evidently, pretreatment denials do reduce utilization, and it is reasonable to conclude that review does increase efficiency by reducing the cost of maintaining dental health.

While pretreatment review has some beneficial effects, relatively few claims are assessed and the explicit net savings from professional denials are only 3 percent of total premiums. Thus, the overall impact of pretreatment review on increasing efficiency is not large. Furthermore, if the indirect costs of the system are included such as costs to patients and dentists, the savings from professional review are reduced further.

Present regulatory systems such as pretreatment review probably have a modest, positive effect on increasing the efficiency of the dental delivery system in producing dental health. Further gains may be made using dental practice profiles to focus on dentists with unusual treatment patterns, possibly associated with inappropriate care. A profile system could reduce the number of claims reviewed and increase the probability that the reviews are focusing on substantial problems.[46] A related approach to improving pretreatment review is the establishment of more effective methods for bringing about changes in the dental practices of "problem" dentists. Under the present system, carriers have few sanctions available to control dentists who habitually overtreat. The usual procedure is denial of payment for the services in question. However, this is a claim-by-claim review, so that denial on one claim does not influence the selection or review of other claims. "Problem" dentists are sometimes known to consultants and special care is taken reviewing their claims, but carriers do not have any legal methods for directly disciplining such providers. Except for rare and difficult-to-prove cases of fraud, dental-insurance carriers depend on high denial rates to bring about the desired changes. For a more effective review system, some insurance-industry leaders have suggested establishing legal relationships with public regulatory agencies.

In the final analysis, it makes little sense to establish a delivery system where a substantial proportion of dentists' treatment decisions are reviewed by other dentists acting as regulatory agents. Such a system is certain to be costly and is unlikely to result in significant increases in efficiency. While it is true, as seen in table 3, that overtreatment exists, most of the costly problems concern crown and bridge services; these services already are closely monitored. Thus, expanding the present review system to examine a larger percentage of claims will be difficult to justify economically. Indeed, in the case of crowns and bridges, savings comparable to those obtained by professional claim reviews could be achieved more efficiently through modification of benefit plans to increase out-of-pocket expenses for these services. Since some expensive services, such as crowns and bridges, involve a large component of personal taste rather than absolute health need, requiring patients to pay a larger proportion of total costs might be the simplest and most efficient solution. The savings could be used to increase utilization of other services that are likely to have greater benefit to the health of insured patients. However, since the marketing impact of such a change in benefit structure is not known, this approach may not be practical.

In conclusion, structural-level regulations probably had an important impact on practice efficiency in the past, but present options may be limited. At the process level, carriers have contractually controlled potentially abused services and have instituted a prospective utilization review system. Evidence suggests that this system does reduce total expenditures, but its effect on efficiency is modest.

Industrial and School-Based Dental Practices

Although groups concerned about rising dental health insurance premiums have the option of establishing their own dental clinics, the previous discussion of nondentist-owned practices suggests that major gains in production efficiency are not a likely result. However, an important variant of the ownership option is locating the dental practice in the work place rather than the surrounding community. Here the issue is not so much ownership but convenient times and places for patient access to dental care.

This section considers the potential efficiency of work- and school-based dental practices. A large proportion of the population is accessible in these locations. Also, industry and schools have a history of providing some health services, making them likely places for dental practices. This section is mostly theoretical because comprehensive evaluations of these types of practices have not been reported.

Industrial dental practices. A substantial fraction of adult Americans spend their work days in large service and manufacturing organizations. If dental-health services are required, employees either schedule an appointment during nonworking hours or leave work to obtain care from community dentists. The first option is often difficult to arrange, because dental services are usually available only during work hours, although the situation is changing in some areas as we saw in Chapter 1. The second option presents employees with another problem. Hourly employees who visit the dentist during work hours have the expenses of lost wages and travel costs in addition to the dental charges. Employers also may incur costs from reduced production efficiency owing to the absence of employees. Opportunity and travel costs are seldom considered in estimates of health-delivery-system efficiency but they could be reduced by locating dental practices in work places.

Placing dental clinics in industrial locations has several other potential advantages worth noting. First, there might be fewer problems with broken or missed appointments. Although there always will be patients who miss appointments, it would be easier in the work place to substitute another patient on short notice. In comparison, most community-based practices have from 5 to 8 percent appointment failure, which probably causes substantial loss of efficiency.[47]

Along with easy access to patients another possible advantage of work-place dental clinics relates to new methods of preventing caries and periodontal disease that involve keeping teeth free of plaque. Mechanical removal of plaque can be achieved through a combination of professional cleanings and conscientious home care. Research in Sweden[48] documented that bringing patients in once every 60 to 90 days to have professionals reinforce proper oral hygiene and clean teeth can effectively reduce periodontal disease and decay. Dental clinics in the work place could see patients four to ten times each year for 20-minute preventive visits. This could be effective in raising the level of dental health and deserves careful investigation.

Increasing patient access to dental care is also likely to increase utilization and expenditures as more employees receive more care. The often-heard argument that long-term dental expenditures should decrease, once employees reach a maintenance level of care, must be considered cautiously. There is little evidence to suggest that multiple visits for preventive care are any cheaper in the long run than episodic visits for curative treatment.

It is too early to tell whether the work place will become a major site for delivering primary health services, as it has become in many countries. Further development will depend, in large part, on the efficiency of these facilities compared to traditional practice systems and their effect on total expenditures, because these are the factors that will presumably motivate employers. It will also depend on employees being willing to substitute relationships with family dentists for the convenience of industrially based dental services.

School dental practices. Providing children with dental care usually requires parents to arrange appointments and accompany children to dental offices. Often this means removing children from school and, because more women work full-time, having a parent take time off. The access problems of single parents who are medically indigent or non-English speaking are even more difficult.

Such problems may be reduced by establishing more school dental clinics where children can receive comprehensive care. School-based dental-delivery systems are common in many nations.

In the United States, especially in urban areas of the Northeast, some public schools have dental operatories used by school hygienists and part-time dentists. Children receive periodic examinations and fluoride treatments from hygienists. Restorative and other treatments performed by dentists are provided to children whose parents are medically indigent or unable to take them to a private dentist. Programs like these often are supported by funds from school or health department budgets.

The advocates of school-based treatment argue that all children, regardless of family income, should be eligible to receive care. However, a comprehensive school-based dental program with universal entitlement is likely to be very low on the agenda of possible new public programs over the next decade or more.[49] Thus, this section concentrates on possible improvements in the delivery system for medically indigent children where the state has already accepted varying degrees of responsibility.

Expansion of school-based dental clinics in the U.S. has been limited by lack of funds and opposed by the dental profession.[50] The funding problem remains the major issue. Most schools lack dental facilities and would face large initial capital outlays for renovations, equipment, and supplies. Operating costs of a dental program also are substantial.

Dental Medicaid programs for the medically indigent offer a partial solution to the funding problem in schools where the majority of children are eligible for Medicaid. The difficulty of raising money for renovations and equipment remain, but in schools with dental facilities, dentists can be employed to provide care, and the school or dentists can bill the Medicaid system to cover the operating costs of the program. Because children eligible for Medicaid often are in special need of dental services, school-based dental programs offer an attractive alternative delivery site for this segment of the population.

Dental profession opposition appears to relate mainly to the establishment of a large public dental-delivery system that would compete with the private sector. The profession's argument is that a large publicly owned and operated medical-care delivery system is alien to the philosophy and traditions of providing health services in the United States. Also deserving consideration is the argument that it would require a major investment in public funds to establish such a system, and that these funds might be more efficiently used by having private sector firms deliver the care.

One alternative might be to allow private dental firms to contract with school boards to provide care in schools with large numbers of Medicaid-eligible children. The capital investment needed to construct, equip, and staff the clinics could be the responsibility of the dental firms, so that public funds would not be required. With (say) a five-year contract, the dental firms could recover their initial investment and operating costs. Depending on the level and structure of fees in the Medicaid program, this approach could be financially feasible. Monitoring for quality also could be far easier than with dispersed private practices. Of equal importance, it is within the framework of the private delivery system and should receive professional support.

In terms of efficiency, school-based private dentistry would have the same advantages already mentioned for industrially-based clinics —namely, fewer missed appointments and increased feasibility of periodic visits for preventive care. Indeed, if the private dental firms were paid a rate per child rather than fees for service, they might have greater incentives to establish effective preventive programs. The increased use of self- and professionally applied topical fluorides, sealants, and cleanings could have a dramatic effect on reducing tooth decay in children.

Most existing Medicaid programs have so many benefit restrictions on the utilization of preventive services (e.g., type of service and frequency of application) that it is financially difficult to support an effective preventive program. A capitation payment system might solve this problem and should entice private dental firms to make the investments needed to establish school-based dental clinics.

A variant on the aforementioned plan would have part or all of the clinic owned by the school system or some other local authority and call for bids from competing dental firms to operate the system for periods of time. While this might lower entry costs for competing bidders, it would raise the capital investment required from public funds, which might cause difficulty.

A final school-based innovation might substantially improve dental care for poor people without much disturbance to the present system. Only inspection would take place at the school; students' families would be contacted subsequently by community-based dentists who would inform them of the needed treatment and their Medicaid entitlement status. Singling out the Medicaid-eligible for inspections presumably would be no more objectionable than school-based treatment. But the latter consideration suggests a broader function for the school-based inspections. After parental consent was gained, all children might be inspected and the information turned over the the designated family dentists who could then contact the parents. No evidence is available on the efficacy of this two-step system for either (1) poor children only or (2) all children where most of them must pay standard fee-for-service rates. However, in the province of Manitoba, Canada, a universal capitation scheme of this kind has claimed treatment rates that rival those of entirely school-based systems.[51]

In conclusion, the location of dental practices in industrial settings and schools theoretically could increase efficiency as a result of: (1) reducing appointment failures; (2) possibly allowing the implementation of preventive programs that require multiple short visits; and (3) decreasing opportunity and travel costs associated with visits to community dental offices during work or school time. They have the disadvantage of fragmenting family dental care among several providers. They could well increase total expenditures for care.

Patient Strategies

For noninsured patients, strategies for increasing efficiency of dental care relate mainly to gaining knowledge of dental disease and treatments, so as to become more efficient consumers. Cost-conscious people can seek out dentists who have low fees but provide care of adequate quality. Citizens, fiscal intermediaries, and financiers of dental care can act through the political system to change laws and regulations that govern dentistry. Presumably, legal changes might lead to increased efficiency in the delivery of dental care.

Patients who have at least some dental insurance can act through their employers, unions, or carriers to increase dental-practice efficiency by the mechanisms previously cited. They can also attempt to decrease their out-of-pocket costs by finding dentists who will accept insurance reimbursement as payment in full for coinsured services. This practice is a source of considerable current controversy between insurers and some dentists; key legal issues remain to be settled.

Dental health legislation. Although they have not had dental care as their essential focus, attempts to reduce the tax advantages of health insurance have recently received a great deal of attention. Most economists and policy analysts ascribe a large part of the explosion of health-care costs in recent years to health insurance. The increase in insurance is attributed largely to its status as untaxed income by the federal government. In response there have been proposals to eliminate or significantly reduce the tax advantages for health insurance. The proposal put forward by Enthoven (see the Introduction to this book) has perhaps the greatest political appeal. It calls for an income-related tax credit, but limited to insurance for a certain package of health services. If dental-insurance premiums were to be considered taxable income, the present growth of dental insurance would certainly slow dramatically or even be reversed. Problems of cost containment that now stem from the absence of patient and practitioner attention to the patient's out-of-pocket costs clearly would be reduced.

Discount dental practices. With the advent of prepayment plans, some dentists have formed practices (or practice associations) that accept the carrier's reimbursement for coinsured services as payment in full. The patient's portion is not collected and is therefore "discounted." Such practices typically offer unusually low prices to uninsured patients as well.

Discount dental practices have been able to reduce their prices by 20 to 50 percent. Since there is little reason to believe that the low unit prices result from technical production efficiencies associated with more effective use of technology or personnel—although this possibility cannot be ruled out—other explanations have been offered.

The discount practices may: (1) employ newly graduated, foreign, semiretired, or other categories of dentists who are willing to accept lower incomes; (2) provide lower-quality services; or (3) increase the services provided per patient, which increases total expenditures even though unit prices are reduced. These strategies are not mutually exclusive.

An unpublished report[52] on one group of discount dental offices suggests that, in part, the third approach is used, i.e., expenditures per patient are significantly higher in discount compared to full-fee practices. If this finding is supported in future studies, the clinical necessity of the additional services would be at issue. While patient demand is expected to increase with reduced out-of-pocket expenses, the possibility exists of dentist-induced demand that does not contribute to improved dental health. Further research is therefore needed to determine if discount practices reduce the unit cost of services while increasing the cost of producing dental health by over-treatment.

It is important to emphasize that this discussion is not meant to imply that all dentists who advertise or discount their fees are unethical or provide inadequate care. However, it may be that dentists initially attracted to these competitive practices are not "mainstream" dentists and represent a fringe group within the profession. Perhaps, as these practices become more established, the majority of dentists will participate, making the dental market more competitive without affecting the quality of care.

DISCUSSION AND CONCLUSIONS

This section briefly expands on some of the major issues previously raised and compares the different strategies for improving the efficiency of the dental delivery system. To start, consideration is given to methods for reducing the cost of services and the cost of producing health; concluding remarks focus on controlling total dental expenditures.

Unit Cost of Service

It does not appear that the methods discussed for influencing provider or payer behavior offer any substantial advantages for reducing the cost of producing dental services. This means that dramatic reductions in the rate of production cost increases are unlikely even as group practices, nondentist-owned practices, and capitation payment plans become more common despite probable increases in price competition. The present delivery system may be reasonably cost-efficient in its use of available resources compared to legal alternatives.

Major reductions in dental costs will probably depend, in the long run, on the development of new technologies to prevent and treat dental diseases. Certainly, the past 20 years have seen important advances in efficiency with the use of high-speed drills and new dental materials. Whether additional gains of similar or greater magnitude are possible remains to be seen, but there is clearly need for more clinical and basic science research.

The feasibility of using expanded function auxiliaries (EFDAs) to perform reversible procedures has received considerable attention, but as noted by Douglass and Lipscomb,[53] EFDAs might have limited immediate impact in private-practice dentistry even if they were legally available. This is because the effective use of EFDAs appears to require a commitment to substantial revision of dental-practice organization which, in turn, is attractive to only a limited number of practitioners. Douglass and Lipscomb thus believe that even without legal strictures, the potential productivity increases from use of EFDAs would only slowly work their way into the mainstream of dentistry. Once again, greater competition among dentists could change the situation considerably by providing a greater stimulus to cost reduction.

The use of auxiliaries to do nonreversible procedures also has been discussed but is not likely, at least in the near future. The dental profession has successfully prevented the development of this type of auxiliary in almost all industrialized countries.

Finally, it may be possible to reduce costs under third-party payment by providing dentists with incentives to work faster so that it takes less time to produce a unit of service. To a large extent the fee-for-service payment system already offers such an incentive; further reductions in treatment times might require government-regulated fixed-fee payment systems. As an example, dentists in the British National Health Service are paid under a fee-for-service system with fees set to allow the average dentist to achieve a government-established target income. Over the years, this system has resulted in low dental fees. To maintain reasonable incomes, British dentists have to produce many services per unit time. However, the increased productivity also may result in lower quality of care and dentist job satisfaction. The effectiveness of this type of control depends on the importance of the third-party payer employing it to the total practice income of the dentist.

One key issue in assessing the value of this productivity strategy for reducing costs is the poorly understood relationship between quality of care and dental health. It is at least conceivable that by some reduction in the quality of care, unit costs could be decreased without decreasing dental health. This is sure to be a central issue if public and private payers attempt to force dental fees down to the point where dentists are required to substantially reduce their treatment times while trying to achieve expected incomes. Of course, it is also possible that payers may hope to reduce dental incomes as well as fees. (See the discussion on rates of return in Chapter 4.)

Costs of Producing Dental Health

Major gains in the efficiency of producing dental health are possible as clinical researchers provide practitioners more data on the effectiveness of specific services and service patterns. Also, the twenty-year national investment in basic dental research is now beginning to pay off with new preventive and therapeutic methods that are more effective than existing treatments. It is the establishment of new technologies rather than changes in the delivery system per se that may offer the greatest potential for efficiencies in generating dental health.

New preventive and therapeutic methods may require major changes in the delivery system. For example, the development of an antiplaque agent that requires quarterly professional applications could result in a major restructuring of benefit plans, practice organizations, and dental education. The present systems for delivering dental care (and medical care) were established to deal with acute illness, not chronic diseases and certainly not prevention. Emphasis on the control of chronic diseases plus the development of new therapies may give major advantages to large practice organizations that can finance and administer the auxiliary personnel and equipment needed to provide low-cost, periodic preventive treatments to large groups of people over extended periods at convenient locations.

Controlling Total Expenditures

The last issue that requires discussion is the problem of controlling total expenditures. Some payer demands for greater efficiency have as their ultimate goal reducing total expenditures. Conflicting with this social goal is the opposing trend to make care more accessible to the disadvantaged, which will undoubtedly lead to greater utilization and expenditures. The resolution of this conflict may be one of the primary social issues of this coming decade. The public needs to be made aware of the fact that even with major gains in delivery-system efficiency and lower prices, total expenditures are likely to increase as more people receive comprehensive, preventively oriented dental care.

At present dentistry has relatively low priority in public and private health expenditures. The reasons for this are several but mainly reflect general attitudes about the importance of dental health compared to other health problems and human services. These attitudes will not be easily changed. As the national effort to control total health costs continues, dentistry may be swept along with social legislation to limit expenditures for medical care. As previously noted, tax subsidies for dental insurance could well be removed with profound effect on the dental market.

The fundamental problem is that the introduction of more cost-effective methods for improving dental health is likely to increase total expenditures. This is especially true for preventive programs. It can be expected in both private markets and public programs because of the greater perceived effectiveness of treatment. The often-heard argument against the implementation of some preventive programs is that their costs equal or exceed the cost of treatment. This position misses the point that preventive programs reduce the incidence of disease and thereby result in more health being produced for the money. If the only criterion for judging the value of innovative methods to improve dental health is total expenditures, there may be little opportunity for significant improvements in the dental-care delivery system.

In conclusion, the application of existing technology to the prevention and treatment of dental disease will probably continue to require funds in at least the same proportion of total health expenditures as is now the case. Some advances in delivery-system efficiency can be expected, but these advances are unlikely to limit, to any substantial degree, public and private expenditures for dental care.

Notes

1. *Distribution of Dentists in the United States by State, Region, District, and County, 1979*, Chicago, American Dental Association, 1979, p. 61.

2. *The 1977 Survey of Dental Practice*, Chicago, American Dental Association, 1978, p. 7; "JADA Association Reports: An Analysis of Dental Practice from 1952 to 1976," *Journal of the American Dental Association*, 100(1):89-98, 1980.

3. C. W. Douglass, and K. D. Nash, "A Comparison of Productivity and Efficiency in Solo and Group Dental Practices." Unpublished manuscript, 1980.

4. D. L. Drier, "Department Store Dental Practices," *American Dental Association News*, February 19, 1979, p. 6.

5. L. R. Punch, "Union Health Center is an Old Hand at Dentistry," *American Dental Association News*, March 24, 1980, pp. 4-5.

6. "Dental Care in Federally Qualified HMOs," *Journal of the American Dental Association*, 99:672-96, 1979.

7. M. H. Schoen, and M. N. Raskin, Personal Communication, 1979.

8. *The 1977 Survey of Hospital Dental Departments*, Chicago, American Dental Association, 1978. p. 17.

9. R. M. Gibson, "National Health Expenditures, 1978," *Health Care Financing Review*, 1(1):1-36, 1979.

10. *The 1977 Survey of Dental Practice*, p. 7.

11. Douglass and Nash, "A Comparison of Productivity."

12. J. E. Kushman, R. Scheffler, L. Miners, and C. Mueller, "Nonsolo Dental Practice: Incentives and Returns to Size," *Journal of Economics and Business*, 31(1):29-39, 1978.

13. J. E. Kushman, and C. F. Nuckton, "Further Evidence on Incentives and Returns to Size in Dental Practice," paper presented at the Western Economic Association, Honolulu: 1978.

14. J. E. Kushman, "Participation of Private Practice Dentists in Medicaid," *Inquiry*, XV:225-33, 1978. For a more detailed discussion of such scale economies, see Chapter 1.

15. R. M. Bailey, "Economics of Scale in Medical Practice," *Empirical Studies in Health Economics*, ed., H. E. Klarman. Baltimore: Johns Hopkins Press, 1970, pp. 255-73. N. Ross, "Impact of the Organization of Practice on Quality of Care and Physician Productivity," *Medical Care*, 18(4):347-59, 1980. H. S. Luft, "Trends in Medical Care Costs: Do HMOs Lower the Rate of Growth?" *Medical Care*, 18(1):1-16, 1980. H. S. Luft, "How do HMOs Achieve Their Savings? Rhetoric and Evidence," *New England Journal of Medicine*, 298(24): 1336-43, 1978.

16. M. H. Schoen, "Dental Care and the Health Maintenance Organization Concept," *Milbank Memorial Fund Quarterly (Health and Society)*, 53(2):173-93, 1975.

17. D. B. Dutton, and R. S. Silber, "Children's Health Outcomes in Six Different Ambulatory Care Delivery Systems," *Medical Care*, 18(7):693-714, 1980; G. T. Perkoff, L. Kahn, and P. Haas, "The Effects of Experimental Prepaid Group Practice on Medical Care Utilization and Cost," *Medical Care*, 14:432-49, 1976; A. A. Scitovsky, L. Benham, and N. McCall, "Use of Physician Services Under Two Prepaid Plans," *Medical Care*, 17(5):441-60, 1979; S. Rhee, "Factors Determining the Quality of Physician Performance in Patient Care," *Medical Care*, 14:733-37, 1976; K. Clute, *The General Practitioner*. Toronto, University of Toronto Press, 1963.

18. D. Conrad, A. P. Milgrom, and A. Dolan. *Assessment of Antitrust Actions Affecting Dentistry: Final Report*, Washington, D.C.: Department of Health, Education, and Welfare, Publication (DMA) 80-20, 1980, p. 33.

19. There is reason to believe that financing problems for a large capitation practice might be quite difficult, however. See Penny S. Elliott, "Dentist-Entrepreneur Creates Expansive Capitation Empire," *Dental Economics*, September, 1980, p. 83.

20. A few states also limit the number of offices a dentist may own. For a discussion, see Chapter 1.

21. M. M. Marcus, and L. J. Drabek, *Study: VA Dental Manpower Requirements: Final Report of National Academy of Sciences contract number ALS34-75-125*, Los Angeles: University of California, 1976.

22. Douglass and Nash, "A Comparison of Productivity", Kushman et al., "Nonsolo Dental Practice."

23. A. Jong, and D. H. Leverett, "The Operation of A Community Dental Clinic in a Health Center: An Evaluation," *Journal of Public Health Dentistry* 31(1):27-31, 1971.

24. Jan Erik Ahlberg, "Dental Care Delivery in Sweden," in John I. Ingle and Patricia Blair, eds., *International Dental Care Delivery Systems* (Cambridge, Mass.: Ballinger Publishing Company, 1978), p. 141.

25. Neville Doherty and Ifkhar Hussain, "Costs of Providing Dental Services for Children in Public and Private Practices," *Health Services Research* 10 (Fall, 1975), pp. 244-53; N. Doherty, P. Horowitz, and G. Crakes, "Real Costs of Dental Care in Private and Public Practices," *Medical Care*, 18(1):96-105, 1980.

26. G. Sparer, and A. Anderson, "Cost of Services at Neighborhood Health Centers: A Comparative Analysis," *New England Journal of Medicine*, 286(23):1241-45, 1972.

27. It must be remembered, however, that part of the independent dentists' real income comes from the quality of their work days; they are not assumed to maximize money profits at the expense of all other considerations. This implies that they may take part of their income in leisure or in the avoidance of the supervision of others. But the price in money income that they pay for these proclivities is higher and more immediate than the price paid by salaried personnel.

28. In fact there may be a trade-off between income and ethical probity. Where on this trade-off locus a practitioner actually works may be heavily determined by his ease of earning income. See R. G. Evans, "Modelling the Objectives of the Physician" in R. Fraser, ed., *Health Economics Symposium: Proceedings of the First Canadian Conference* (Kingston, Ontario: Queens University Industrial Relations Centre, 1976); R. G. Evans and M. F. Williamson, *Extending Canadian Health Insurance: Pharmacare and Denticare* (Toronto: Ontario Economic Council, 1978), Frank Sloan and Roger Feldman, "Monopolistic Elements in the Market for Physician Services," paper presented at Federal Trade Commission Conference, June 1, 1977.

29. C. R. Buck, and K. L. White, "Peer Review: Impact of a System Based on Billing Claims," *New England Journal of Medicine*, 291:877-83, 1974; E. Faltermayer, "Where Doctors Scramble for Patients' Dollars," *Fortune*: November 6, 1978, 114-20.

30. Douglass and Nash, "A Comparison of Productivity and Efficiency"; Kushman et al., "Nonsolo Dental Practice."

31. Robert T. Kudrle, "Dental Care," in Judith Feder, John Holahan, and Theodore Marmor, eds., *National Health Insurance: Conflicting Goals and Policy Choices* (Washington, D.C.: The Urban Institute, 1980), p. 578; Helen Avnet and M. Nikias, *Insured Dental Care* (New York: Group Health Dental Insurance, Inc., 1967).

32. H. L. Bailit, Third Party Quality Assurance Systems, Final Report of Grant Number HS01824, Hyattsville, MD: National Center for Health Services Research, Department of Health, Education, and Welfare, 1980.

33. H. L. Bailit, "Issues in Regulating Quality of Care and Containing Costs Within Private Sector Policy," *Journal of Dental Education*, in press.

34. M. H. Schoen, "Group Practice in Dentistry," *Medical Care*, 5(3):176-83, 1967.

35. M. H. Schoen, "Observation of Selected Dental Services Under Two Prepayment Mechanisms," *American Journal of Public Health*, 63:727-31, 1973.

36. H. M. Rosen, R. A. Sussman, and E. J. Sussman, "Capitation in Dentistry: A Quasi-Experimental Evaluation," *Medical Care*, 15(3):228-40, 1977.

37. G. L. Cogan, "A Quantitative Comparison of Services Performed for Fee-for-Service and Capitation Patients," *Journal of the American Dental Association*, 91(4):836-37, 1975.

38. E. D. Olsen, & G. F. Chetelat, "Dental Capitation Program: A Comparison of Delivery Systems," *California Dental Association Journal*, 55:47-50, 1979.

39. Luft, "How do HMOs Achieve Their Savings?"

40. W. J. Gies, *Dental Education in the United States and Canada: A Report to the Carnegie Foundation for the Advancement of Teaching*, New York: The Carnegie Foundation, 1926.

41. See, for example, "Survey of Attitudes on Dental Licensing Procedures," *Journal of the American Dental Association*, 85(6):1270, 1972.

42. S. T. Reisine, and H. L. Bailit, "History and Organization of Pretreatment Review, A Dental Utilization Review System," *Public Health Reports*, 95(3):282-90, 1980.

43. H. L. Bailit, M. Raskin, S. Reisine, and D. Chiriboga, "Controlling the Cost of Dental Care," *American Journal of Public Health*, 69(7):699-703, 1979.

44. H. L. Bailit, unpublished data, 1979.

45. H. L. Bailit, unpublished data, 1979.

46. H. L. Bailit, and J. Clive, "The Development of Dental Practice Profiles," *Medical Care*, 19:30-46, 1981.

47. J. G. DiStasio, "The Occurrence of 'No Show' Appointments Among Medicaid and Private Dental Patients," *Journal of the Massachusetts Dental Society*, 18:82, 1969.

48. P. Axelsson, and J. Lindhe, "Effect of Controlled Oral Hygiene Procedures on Caries and Periodontal Disease in Adults," *Journal of Clinical Periodontology*, 5(2):133-51, 1978.

49. For an evaluation of alternative options for broader entitlement, see Kudrle, "Dental Care."

50. R. C. Warren, and E. Potts, *School-Based Dental Delivery Systems*, Washington, D.C.: Public Health Service, in press.

51. Robert T. Kudrle, "Foreign Lessons for Dental Coverage Under U.S. National Health Insurance," *Journal of Health Politics, Policy and Law*, Winter 1981.

52. J. L. Kramer, unpublished data, 1979.

53. C. W. Douglass, and J. K. Lipscomb, "Expanded Function Dental Auxiliaries: Potential for the Supply of Dental Services in a National Dental Program," *Journal of Dental Education*, 43(10):556-67, 1979.

3

Auxiliary Personnel

David O. Born

INTRODUCTION

Cost containment in dentistry can be achieved through a variety of techniques. Community water fluoridation can prevent a certain amount of dental disease, eliminate the need for specific types of dental services, and thus restrain dental-care costs. Another way to contain costs is to monitor the delivery of dental services to minimize unnecessary procedures. A third approach seeks to use the lowest-cost method of providing services. This latter approach will be addressed in this chapter.

The central question, then, is this: "Are we providing dental services by the lowest-cost method?" More specifically, do dental auxiliaries offer potential for lowering the cost of services, and, if so, are we likely to reduce costs by utilizing auxiliaries?

For the most part, the phrase "lowest-cost method" refers to explicit costs, i.e., costs of the input factors that are attributed to the production of dental services.

Dentistry, like most other service industries, is labor intensive: labor is the primary input factor. In other words, productivity gains are most directly a function of increasing labor inputs.[1] Some productivity increases have been and will be made possible via capital investment (e.g., high-speed drills), but overall, in the dental sector

The author wishes to acknowledge the assistance of Dr. Robert Evans who contributed both extensively and graciously to the development of this paper. Thoughtful assistance was also provided by Dr. Joseph Lipscomb, Dr. Robert Kudrle and Mr. Ronald Bognore. Appreciation is extended to all of these individuals.

productivity is increased in proportion to (or constrained by) the labor expended by dentists to produce services.

The services provided by the dentist involve the evaluation of dental health and the performance of certain procedures intended to prevent dental disease or restore and maintain dental health and appearance. Virtually all dental procedures consist of clearly defined tasks, each of which requires a specific level of skill, manual dexterity, and informed judgment.

It has long been known that some of the component tasks could be delegated to persons other than the dentist.[2] In fact, the first dental assistants appeared with the emergence of dentistry as a profession in the mid-1800s. The first auxiliaries "received patients, performed 'housekeeping' chores and handled clerical and bookkeeping procedures." Later, they began to assist dentists in treating patients.

Dental hygienists were first trained informally in 1905, in Connecticut, where a formal program was established in 1913. Their primary responsibilities have always been to provide dental prophylactic care, although, in the opinion of many educators, the scope and depth of their training, particularly since the sixties, qualifies them to perform additional duties. Like dental assistants, dental laboratory technicians date back to the 1850s. They do the work required to develop prosthetic devices for dental patients, and they generally work in dental laboratories or for individual dentists.

Because auxiliaries are able to substitute their labor for that of the dentist in performing certain dental tasks, and because labor costs for auxiliaries are lower than those for dentists, it is obvious that auxiliary labor represents a potential avenue for cost containment. As productivity is increased (or if productivity is held constant when nonlabor costs are rising), reduction of labor costs through substitution may provide a stabilizing or cost-containing function.

Because the dental profession has been using auxiliaries in some fairly traditional ways for many years, attention here will focus primarily on two substitution options that have been presented to dentistry over the past two decades. The first of these is the denturist, the second is the Expanded Function Dental Auxiliary (EFDA). We will also consider two other auxiliary alternatives: school dental nurses, who with expanded functions are able to work with minimal and indirect supervision; and independent dental hygienists, whose work is a relatively new development not unlike school dental nursing, but which is controversial because it has emerged in defiance of state laws.

DENTURISTS

The term *denturist* refers to a person other than a dentist who provides denture services directly to the public. According to a historical review of denturism,[3] denturists have practiced illegally in the United States and abroad for many years. Advocates of legal recognition have been vocal in recent years, giving rise to what has been called a "denturist movement."

This movement has its roots in Europe, where legislative recognition was first given to dental mechanics in Germany in 1914. In 1952, apparent abuses of the privileges extended to these technicians and their encroachment into "nonmechanical" service areas led to revocation of their right to practice independently. A number of other countries, however, permit dental laboratory technicians (under a variety of titles) to provide dentures (and in some cases, other services) directly to the public.

The closing of the denturist industry in Germany coincided with shortages of dental laboratory technicians in Canada. Recruitment efforts by Canadian laboratory owners led to the emigration of many German denturists to North America. Before long, some of these technicians and their native Canadian counterparts were working directly with the public, independent of licensed dentists. Legislation eventually gave denturists official sanction in eight of the ten Canadian provinces.

Starting in 1955, similar efforts to attain status as independent health-care providers were made by American dental laboratory technicians. While these efforts have been strongly opposed by dentists, a particularly intense flurry of state campaigns in the late seventies resulted in denturist victories in Arizona, Maine and Oregon.

In Arizona and Maine, dentists and denturists settled on compromise positions without taking the issue to the public via the referendum process. The agreements provided for the licensing of denturists and the establishment of educational criteria and training requirements. The new regulations further specified "that a denturist can practice only under the supervision of a licensed dentist."[4]

In Oregon, the issue was taken to the polls. In spite of the fact that both the Oregon and the American Dental Associations waged a bitter media battle with denturist supporters (at a cost of $400,000 to $500,000), 78 percent of the voters approved a referendum that permitted denturists to establish independent practices as of July 1980.

An ADA-sponsored analysis of the Oregon experience points out that while dentists characterized the issue as health-related, the vast majority of voters saw it in economic terms. Fueled by the consumerism movement and an insurgent "anti-professional" attitude, Oregon voters voiced clearly their right to choose how and from whom dentures will be purchased.[5]

The public-opinion survey discussed in the ADA analysis reveals a strong sentiment in favor of reduced health-care costs, a belief that health professionals have controlled the market in their own interest, and a desire to assert individual freedom of choice. The response of organized dentistry in Oregon to the pro-denturists, according to the report, was unprofessional and embarrassing to many dentists; if anything, the campaign tarnished the image of the profession and weakened public confidence in dentists.

The resounding defeat of dentistry's position stunned dentists around the country. It was as though a land mine had been exploded at the very foundation of the profession.

Dentistry had good cause for anxiety. Like other professions, dentistry has been given a societal mandate to provide a specific spectrum of services. As professionals, dentists are given status and privileges. In return they are expected to behave responsibly and ethically. So great has the public's trust been, that the profession has been largely self-regulated and, consequently, it has had monopolistic control over the market as sole provider of a particular range of services.

In Oregon dentistry, in effect, submitted its mandate to the public for a "vote of confidence." To the profession's surprise and dismay, the electorate ignored the dentists' recommendation and extended a portion of that mandate to a previously unlicensed and unrecognized group, the denturists. Furthermore, this new group of providers was given *independent* status, thus preventing dentistry from retaining its monopolistic control of the dental marketplace.

Until the Oregon referendum, dentistry's control had been far-reaching, encompassing admission to dental schools, accreditation of curricula, and domination of state boards of dentistry. Rigid socialization of members to the standards and expectations of the profession had been achieved through long training programs and the pervasive influence of state and national associations in all areas of professional life. Those associations typically claim membership of 85 to 95 percent of the dentists in a given state. In most states, graduates of a handful of dental schools tend to dominate. There is a strong sense of camaraderie within the profession; numerous channels of communication permit an open flow of information at all levels.

Rigid socialization and esprit de corps are critical to this discussion of cost containment because it is through them that control over the profession is maintained and economic self-interest is protected.

Monopoly power rests on the ability to control output. Dentistry, consisting as it does of thousands of small, unrelated firms, cannot control output directly. Instead, the profession is able to use various collective restraints to control the production and licensing of both dentists and auxiliaries. This, in turn, controls the supply of services. Further, if persons trained and admitted to full membership in the profession are sufficiently well socialized, it is unlikely that they will break from the status quo, particularly with respect to the functioning of the dental marketplace. (The prohibition against dental advertising that existed until the late seventies is an example of this point.) Once in practice, dentists as a group profit most when they adopt a "live-and-let-live" attitude. That is, they are expected to take a reasonable share of the market but not to undercut (outproduce or underprice) their fellows.

Evans[6] argues that dentists and other self-employed professionals, such as owner-managers, may not benefit collectively from improved "industry-wide" efficiency. As prices are lowered to sell the increased output that has been made possible by increased efficiency, dentists are faced with the very real possibility of a drop in net profits for all firms. Such a possibility serves as a conscious or unconscious inducement for collective restraints by dentists (and other professionals).

Furthermore, when viewed from the perspective of the individual dentist, increasing efficiency through auxiliary employment may not be particularly attractive since the dentist is likely to *believe* that increased output may not be marketable at a competitive price. In addition, substituting auxiliary time for a dentist's time in the operatory may not be attractive because the *real value* to the dentist of an hour of time saved may not be significant in a comparative sense. Thus, because of the constraints on dental incomes and dental-service sales, *increased efficiency for one dentist in a community cuts into collective incomes of other dentists*. Moreover, unless sizable increases in demand occur, a dentist operating efficiently works to the detriment of his peers. A dynamic resistance is thus created, enabling virtually all dentists (as a collective) to maximize their incomes. The situation is a little like the old union game of "featherbedding."

Evans further explains that the conditions under which auxiliaries are profitable are conditions which make the entire market unstable in that real dental efficiency would induce strong competitive responses, the end result of which would be that all dentists would end up with lower incomes.

Monopolizing the dental economy is possible because dentists, individually and collectively, exercise great control over auxiliaries. They determine how many are trained and how many are hired. While there are modest incentives for some practices to employ some auxiliaries (and thereby achieve more efficient production), it is believed (whether at a conscious or subconscious level) that dentistry as a whole would lose from the enormous increase in production that the widespread use of auxiliaries would make possible.

As long as traditional socialization is maintained and dentists constrain the auxiliary work force, then monopolistic control will continue—as it has in Arizona and Maine. Despite their grousing about a denturist victory, dentists really won the battle there. By working out a compromise in which denturists were given legal status but were required to work under the supervision of dentists, the dentists effectively relegated denturists to employee status.

Ultimately, it is this matter of supervision that is really central to cost containment. A. K. Dolan, in his assessment of Federal Trade Commission actions in dental licensing, notes that if the commission pursues its investigations regarding denturism, the end result is likely to be a "nullification of states' prohibitions against direct patient-denturist relations."[7] The issue then will become one not so much of whether denturists will practice legally, but how denturists will be incorporated into dental delivery systems under state practice acts.

The alternatives cited by Dolan include dental supervision, as in Arizona and Maine; independent practice with dental-health certification by a dentist or physician, as in Oregon; or complete independence with no dental-health certification required.

In states where denturists work under supervision, they are simply employees of the dental firm. While denturists may meet patients face-to-face, it is still the dentist who controls the relationship (including denturist employment) and determines the ultimate acceptability of the product.

Simply having a low-cost labor source available does not guarantee that it will be employed in production. The decision in most states rests with dentists. As we have seen, dentistry's economic self-interest may work against employing auxiliaries.

From an industry-wide perspective, then, regulations permitting supervised use of auxiliaries are not likely to lead to either widespread employment of denturists or to cost containment. But in states where denturists may deal independently with the public and generally function as separate firms, the potential for cost containment exists. As separate firms producing some of the same products as dentists, denturists present a direct competitive threat. The threat to dentistry is all the greater because denturists are not socialized to the same standards and values as dentists; the esprit de corps that exists among denturists is clearly not with dentists. Denturists presently have no commitment to the status quo in dentistry.

Putting questions of power and control aside for a moment, we can say that insofar as denturists provide denture service independently, they represent substitutes for dentists. This "new" input factor has potential for increasing productivity within the dental care field and, depending on the costs of denturist labor, production costs could decline. Denturists typically have less expensive training and a smaller range of skills than dentists, so their labor charges would be lower.

Cost Comparison

Very little data exist on the cost of denturist services compared to the cost of denture services provided by dentists. Recent dental insurance claims information from Ontario shows that the average single denture billing by denturists was $130 compared to $239 by dentists. Fees for full upper and lower dentures were $250 for denturists compared to $435 for dentists. Dental fees for dentures in Ontario increased 66.7 percent between 1974 and 1979, while fees for preventive services rose 125 percent. Such data might lead one to think that competition from denturists had served to contain costs, but fees for restorative services, for which no competitive provider exists, rose only 50 percent.[8] Other data on denturist costs, fees and market impact apparently are nonexistent.[9]

Where denturists have the opportunity to establish independent practices, the matter of cost containment on their part becomes a function of how the evolving "profession" behaves.

Denturists, for the most part, are former dental laboratory technicians. Dental laboratory technicians typically receive their training in a vocational school, in the military, in a dental office, or by working as an apprentice in a dental lab. There is little systematic training and any socialization that occurs usually comes from work experience. While dental laboratory owners, denturists, and denturist-supporters are organized, there is no tightly knit association that can be considered comparable (in terms of power and influence on its members) to the American Dental Association.

Among the issues that will bear watching during the eighties is the manner in which denturists are to be educated and formally organized. One would expect that as regulations governing denturists are put into effect in each state, "grandfather" clauses (exempting current denturists from some rules) will be used to create the initial pool of workers. The founders then will have the option (one way or another) of determining the composition of the profession's future membership, training requirements, and licensure requirements. The cost-containment potential of denturists will hinge on the extent to which these "grandfathered" denturists adopt a controlling posture toward their profession.

Evans suggests that if denturists are to emerge as an effective cost-containment force, there must be a sufficient increase in the number of denturists in practice. ("Sufficient" implies that the pool is large enough so that denturists are forced to compete aggressively among themselves and with dentists.) Furthermore, the regulation of denturists, as well as the costs of training, must be kept flexible (and out of the direct control of dentists) so that rapid and continuing growth of the denturist pool can occur. "If entry to the field is too limited, denturists won't advertise or practice efficiently. They won't go after the low prices to aggressively take business away from dentists. Instead, they'll adopt a "live-and-let-live" policy, setting prices somewhat below those of dentists and thereby taking their share of the [profession's] monopoly gains."[10]

If history is a guide, one would be inclined to believe that denturists will exercise fairly tight control on their membership as soon as they take power in the field. They will do so, probably, for the avowed purpose of ensuring the quality of the product and the health of the public. Nonetheless, denturists can be expected to emerge as a significant dental auxiliary within the next five years. Because the dental profession has adopted public opposition to denturists (and thus will find it difficult to accept compromise regulations), it seems all the more likely that denturists will operate independently of dentistry as it is organized today. Consequently, denturists as independent competitors will serve to help contain costs, although probably only to a nominal degree.

Among the factors that lead to this conclusion are these:

First, the present activities of the Federal Trade Commission (FTC) will, in all likelihood, continue in full force. Sellars has noted that since 1970, several Supreme Court cases have "reduced the formerly impervious right of professions to regulate themselves, either through their associations or through closely-associated state agencies."[11] Commission decisions have provided moral (if not legal) support to FTC investigators who, in their examination of the health-care industry, appear increasingly convinced that the professions have acted chiefly to their own advantage. Sellars explains that many professional practices "may violate laws which prohibit anti-competitive behavior and unfair or deceptive practices. What were previously considered to be sacrosanct professional traditions blending both economic self-interest and public interest become examples of price-fixing, restrictions on market entry, refusals to deal, collusion, and unfair constraints on consumer information."

In terms of the denturist issue, it is worth noting that the FTC's primary objective is to promote competition in the economy. Thus far in their inquiries, little evidence has been mustered to support legal restrictions that inhibit competition by prohibiting denturists from dealing independently with the public.

The FTC investigations couple nicely with growing U.S. consumerism. The public's desire to have more purchase options and a stronger voice in the marketplace shows no sign of weakening. This desire for self-determination as purchasers of goods and services will tend to put consumers on the side of any FTC actions that reach the courts, the media, or the polls.

Senior citizen groups are also likely to support denturism. Senior citizen oganizations were very active in Oregon and won many votes for denturism in the referendum there. The number of senior citizens is increasing, and there is every reason to believe that more legislation addressing the concerns of old people will be passed. The cost and availability of dental services are certainly among the basic concerns of the elderly.

Further support for independent denturism will derive from the evolving socioeconomic environment. Since 1974 the mood of the people has made economic concerns paramount; increasing distrust of "big government" and a sense that the economy is out of control contribute to a deep-seated sense of urgency. There appears to be a widespread feeling that the health professions have been looking out for themselves rather than the public welfare. The notion of an "open mandate" for health professionals is consequently under close scrutiny. As public policy develops over the next few years, one can expect (or hope) that policymakers will be guided by a desire to alleviate economic hardship, win public support, and restore a sense of self-determination to the people. In the evolving socioeconomic climate, the denturist movement should have little difficulty realizing its objectives.

Health Impacts

As a final consideration, it should be noted that the literature on the Canadian denturism experience contains little reference to severe health problems arising in patients treated by denturists. The reports that do exist are anecdotal and lack convicing proof. Much of organized dentistry's argument against denturists rests on the possibility of such health problems. Hard evidence to support the contention that denturists are unqualified and that they present a health hazard to the public has yet to be presented and thus dentistry appears to be raising a moot, if not transparent, point.

Given the trends outlined above, public policy will tend to favor independent denturism and there will be modest cost-containment benefits arising from its expansion. From a political perspective, one might suggest that the dental profession examine its motives for opposing the denturist movement.

If the opposition truly stems from a concern about public health, then the profession should move to recommend training and licensure standards that would safeguard individual dental health and not be overly restrictive.

If, on the other hand, the opposition is motivated by a perceived economic threat, then actions, such as those taken in Arizona and Maine, where denturists were incorporated or co-opted into the system, would seem more advantageous to dentistry than those in Oregon where the profession apparently succeeded in portraying itself in unpopular opposition to inexpensive dental care for the elderly.

EXPANDED FUNCTION DENTAL AUXILIARIES: HYGIENISTS' ASSISTANTS

Despite the long history of auxiliaries in dentistry, widespread use of auxiliaries is a relatively recent phenomenon. In the case of dental hygienists, it cannot yet be said to be commonplace.

Data from the American Dental Association show that in 1952, 56.5 percent of independent, nonsalaried dentists employed a full-time assistant and 6.6 percent employed a full-time hygienist. By 1975, 87.8 percent of independent dentists employed a full-time assistant and 21.8 percent employed a full-time hygienist.[12]

In looking at these figures, we must recall that in the fifties and early sixties, use of auxiliaries was largely a result of increasing demand for dental practices coupled with dentists' recognition that auxiliaries could be used advantageously in the dental office.

The Impact of Management Sciences

At the same time, however, there was a much more pervasive force at work—new management sciences. The impact of these sciences on dentistry, via information presented in journals, magazines, and dental curricula, precipitated some fundamental and irrevocable changes in the dental profession, the consequences of which have yet to be fully realized.

By way of background, Shanks, a British economist and journalist, noted that the American economy in the fifties faced two major challenges. The first was labor costs that were two to three times as high as those in Europe; the second was lethargic consumers. In response to consumer lethargy, tremendous emphasis was placed on the marketing of goods and services. In an effort to cut labor costs, great attention was given to new technology and automation. The ultimate impact of these developments on the economy as a whole was a "great upsurge of interest in the techniques of management."[13]

This upsurge was buoyed by an increasing belief in the power of science. This collective public mood was epitomized by the support given to the space race. With technocracy as the "wave of the future," society saw the emergence of a new cult of management specialists who brought their quantitative skills to bear on the problems of American industry.

Success after success was chalked up by the new managers as they moved from one industry to another. It was only a matter of time before dentistry fell under the spell of their promises of efficiency, increased productivity and profits, and greater employee satisfaction.

Early explorations. The first major impact of the management sciences on dentistry occurred in the late fifties when the Public Health Service initiated a series of pilot programs exploring the training of dental students in how to use assistants to increase productivity. Previous studies had suggested that efficient use of chairside auxiliaries could increase productivity from 30 to 40 percent with the use of one auxiliary and up to 65 percent with the use of two auxiliaries.[14]

In 1961, under a congressional appropriation, dental auxiliary utilization programs were established in all dental schools. In 1964, the Public Health Service founded the Dental Manpower Development Center in Louisville, Kentucky. During the early years at Louisville, special attention was focused on increasing productivity through such devices as the "wheel," which gave the dentist supervisory control over multiple chairs and auxiliaries.

Between 1965 and 1975, dental schools jumped on the management bandwagon. Faculty were hired to teach dental business management and management communications. Efficiency was to be dentistry's savior, and the management sciences were its gospel.

Other forces were at work as well, not the least of which was the

"war on poverty" and the hope it engendered among people at all
levels of society that at least some of our social problems might be
solved. Health care was one such problem and in the sixties, many
people held to the conviction that we were moving toward a healthier
society.

So it was during the sixties, while dentists were becoming aware
of the advantages of using auxiliaries and improving their business
management, that dental leaders, government planners, and dental
educators looked to the future and saw an impending dental-care
crisis: the population was expanding more rapidly than the supply
of dental services.[15] A consensus existed that unless measures were
taken to increase the delivery capacity of the profession, substantial
numbers of people would be underserved.

In response to the anticipated crisis, additional dental schools were
constructed, enrollments were expanded, curricula were shortened
and the number of auxiliary programs was increased greatly between
1963 and 1976. It is particularly important to recall as well that the
influence of the management mystique was continuing during this
period. Considerable resources were devoted, through research and
teaching, to increasing management efficiency in dental offices and
developing the use of a "new" assistant, the Expanded Function
Dental Auxiliary (EFDA).

The EFDA concept was sanctioned, if not spawned, by manage-
ment-systems thinking and was recognized by many people as a
"technological breakthrough" that reduced the human capital necessary to provide dental care. Because auxiliaries were trained to perform an expanded role, their ability to serve as labor substitutes was
distinctly greater than that of traditional instrument-handling assistants. In a number of experimental programs, expanded-function
dental auxiliaries were trained to cut cavity preparations and to place
and carve restorations. These particular functions greatly increased
the potential impact of auxiliaries on the production process.[16]

Virtually every study examining these new aides between 1963
and 1976 documented the economic viability of EFDAs.[17] The studies all reported increases in productivity (up to 400 percent, depending on the size and configuration of the dental team). The Louisville
Dental Manpower Development Center, for example, reported that a
dentist working with four EFDAs could increase productivity by 133
percent over a dentist working with a single chairside assistant. The
studies also reported big increases in potential income (up to 169
percent, depending on the size and configuration of the dental team).
The quality of EFDA restorative work was consistently found to be

at least equal to that of dentists, and patients reported high levels of satisfaction.[18]

Six studies[19] looked at dental-service costs once again in the mid-1970s, and the authors were unanimous in identifying cost reduction as a benefit to be gained from use of EFDAs. The cost reductions obtained for restorations, on a unit basis, ranged from 6 to 50 percent. No study found EFDAs to be a more expensive method of delivering care.

In addition to these studies, all of which were clinical in nature, there was considerable exploration of the effect of EFDAs in dental offices and clinics by means of computer simulation.

Kilpatrick's work at Florida[20] and the work at Case Western Reserve[21] are among the best-known studies, but much unpublished work was also carried out at the University of Toronto, the University of Alabama, the University of Pennsylvania, the University of Minnesota, and elsewhere.

These studies (with the exception of Minnesota's) were generally based on mathematical, optimizing models such as those developed at Florida and Case Western Reserve. Following accepted modeling procedures adopted from the fields of economics, engineering, and operations research, investigators examined various input factors, manipulated team configurations, looked at output indicators, and identified optimal personnel mixes.

The approach used at Minnesota could be termed "logistical" in that the computer model used actual patient treatment plans, "real time" schedules, and office-based heuristics (scheduling decision rules)[22] rather than "twice removed" mathematical functions, standardized estimates, and probability distributions.

Both the optimizing and logistical approaches were used to evaluate the efficiency and efficacy of team configurations; both reached similar conclusions. Productivity could be increased and costs reduced through the use of EFDAs. (One especially important point, however, is the scope of functions that can be delegated. Lipscomb and Scheffler, using a linear programming model for resource allocation, found that the "costs of [various] legal restrictions on the [expanded function dental auxiliaries] are high." Also, "output does not increase as much as total cost with the introduction of restrictions."[23] Similarly, the work performed at Minnesota and Florida[24] showed that if the expanded functions did not include placing and carving restorations, the impact of auxiliaries on productivity and costs was considerably reduced. Allowing auxiliaries to cut hard tissue greatly enhanced productivity. The determining factor in estimating potential productivity is the extent to which auxiliaries are dependent on the dentist to participate in some portion of patient treatment. When auxiliaries can independently perform entire restorative procedures, the greatest gains are possible).

Whether the work was clinical or simulated, however, there was no escaping the influence of management science and operations research. This influence, as has been noted, was an outgrowth of the systems thinking that was in vogue in the early sixties and the popularity of management science in the business community. Much of this "new" science was, in turn, made possible by the increased availability of computer technology.[25]

Forces converge. During the sixties and the seventies, dentistry witnessed the convergence of several socioeconomic forces that left an indelible imprint on the profession. The early utilization of auxiliary personnel was a logical response to growing demand. The response "caught on" and was further amplified, expanded, and sanctified by the management mystique. In retrospect, we can see these key influences at work:

An evangelistic movement of systems analysts, operations researchers, efficiency experts, and management technologists.

A desire within organized dentistry to shake the "cottage-industry" image and create a new, modern image.

An anticipated health-care delivery crisis in the wings.

Encouragement from organized dentistry and the federal government to experiment with new delivery techniques.

As these influences worked their way through dentistry, people looked for developments holding the most promise for re-creating the dental profession as a modern (i.e., efficient, well-organized, highly productive, integrated) component in the health-care sector.

Group practice, dental-health maintenance organizations, and the expansion of third-party payment systems were all tested and found promising. But not surprisingly, Expanded Function Dental Auxiliaries were seen as the key to dentistry's future. Thus one study group concluded that EFDAs were "confident in their ability to perform expanded functions; that dentist-employers were highly satisfied with the training and competence of their EFDAs; that EFDAs do stimulate greater efficiency and productivity in many different types of dental practices and receive greater earnings as a result; and that the typical dental patient is willing to receive, and is satisfied with, dental care provided by the dental practices that utilize EFDAs."[26]

In the context of management science as applied to dentistry, R. A. Hankin stated that "The need for efficiency requires that all personnel are allowed to utilize their productive capabilities to the fullest extent. It is not sufficient that any given task be carried out efficiently; it must be delegated to the proper personnel. If two individuals—a physician (or dentist) and an allied health worker, for example—are both equally capable of carrying out a given task, economic efficiency dictates that the least costly individual be delegated the tasks. To do otherwise would be to waste scarce resources—in this instance the physician's (or dentist's) time—which should be used in performing those functions which cannot be delegated."[27]

C. W. Douglass and J. M. Day, after examining the cost-effectiveness of auxiliaries in providing dental services, concluded that "dental auxiliaries in both traditional and extended function modes have significant potential for holding down program costs." They further argued that "the potential for the greater cost-effective use of expanded function dental auxiliaries is clearly available as an alternative for making more dental services available to more people at the same time avoiding significant cost escalation."[28]

Despite what appeared to economists and managers to be overwhelming proof of the cost-effectiveness of EFDAs, the new health workers were not welcomed by a majority of the profession. In fact, dental educators and government officials were stung by a sharp backlash in the late seventies. Expanded function auxiliary programs in at least two states were closed under pressure from state dental boards and state dental associations, and many other programs were modified or curtailed.

Milgrom and Conrad[29] have traced American Dental Association resolutions on EFDAs through the sixties and seventies, pointing out in the process how the profession drew back, in the late seventies, from what had been a fairly progressive posture on delegation of functions. While the historical circumstances surrounding dentistry over the past twenty years are sufficiently complicated as to defy tidy explanation, the end result of the productivity and efficiency "push" between 1960 and 1976 was a dental industry that was technologically (and psychologically) geared up for a massive demand that failed to materialize;[30] in other words, there was rapid growth in the supply of dentists while demand for dental care failed to increase as rapidly as expected.

Professional resistance. With the recession of 1974 and the subsequent decline in dental demand, the profession began to feel overextended in its delivery capability. In reaction, the ax fell heaviest on expanded function programs. (Dental school enrollments stood second in line.)

Thus, after fifteen years of official policy favoring auxiliary utilization and experimentation, the ADA House of Delegates (a policy-making body) passed this resolution in 1975:

Resolved, that the American Dental Association oppose the preparation of teeth, the placement, carving and contouring of dental restorations . . . by dental auxiliaries, and be it further

Resolved, that final decisions related to dental practice and utilization of dental auxiliaries rest with the state society and the state board of dentistry . . ."[31]

But even though the profession turned its back on EFDAs, their potential for cost-containment has not been overlooked by policy-makers. In March 1980, the Comptroller General's office filed a Report to the Congress. The title of the report leaves little doubt as to the conclusions reached by researchers in the General Accounting Office (GAO): *Increased Use of Expanded Function Dental Auxiliaries Would Benefit Consumers, Dentists, and Taxpayers.*[32]

The GAO document provides an overview of dentistry and its manpower resources, presents evidence of the need for more accessible and affordable dental care, and reviews the literature on EFDAs. As we noted earlier, a review of the literature leads one to conclude that EFDAs can provide high-quality, low-cost dental services, including dental restorations.

The GAO analysts reached the following conclusions:

Employing EFDAs for completing restorations benefits both consumers and dentists by increasing the efficiency and effectiveness of the dental-care delivery system.

Extensive research clearly and conclusively shows that EFDAs can be trained to complete high-quality restorations, under the dentists' supervision, without any adverse effect or impact on patients. Research has also shown that employing EFDAs in this manner significantly increases a dentist's productivity.

Dentists already employing EFDAs in this manner said it enabled them to (1) serve more patients, (2) devote additional time to more complicated procedures, and (3) provide higher quality dental care. Some dentists also stated that using EFDAs to complete restorations enabled them to reduce their dental fees.

Interestingly, the tone of the GAO conclusions is tempered by recognition of the present-day political reality of dentistry, a reality that emerged with the 1975 ADA resolution against EFDAs.

In an effort to reconsider that position, the ADA convened a workshop on EFDAs in 1976. Some 260 dentists, educators, researchers, and policymakers examined and discussed the well-worn evidence. After the workshop, the ADA Council on Dental Education and the ADA Board of Trustees recommended to the House of Delegates that the 1975 ADA resolution be rescinded.

As might have been expected from a reading of the mood of professional dentistry at the time, the delegates continued their opposition to EFDAs and stated as their rationale a belief that "effective and safe performance is dependent upon making judgments that require synthesis and application of knowledge acquired in professional dental education."[33] The ADA policy opposing EFDAs remained in force through the 1980 annual session.

The GAO recognizes that the ADA resolution is not binding on state dental boards and lawmakers. It is in state laws, the GAO notes, that one finds the real barriers to increasing the productivity of the nation's dental-care delivery system.

Members of Congress (the GAO's target audience) undoubtedly are aware that state practice acts determine who may provide dental

Table 1. States in Which the Dental Practice Act Gives Authority
to the Board of Dentistry to Delegate Expanded Functions
to Dental Hygienists or Dental Assistants

Arizona	Montana
Arkansas	Nebraska
California	Nevada
Colorado	New Hampshire
Connecticut	New Jersey
Delaware	New Mexico
Florida	North Carolina
Georgia	Ohio
Hawaii	Oklahoma
Idaho	Oregon
Indiana	Pennsylvania
Kansas	Rhode Island
Kentucky	South Carolina
Louisiana	South Dakota
Maine	Tennessee
Maryland	Texas
Massachusetts	Vermont
Michigan	Virginia
Minnesota	West Virginia
Mississippi	Wisconsin
Missouri	Wyoming

Source: Comptroller General, *Increased Use of Expanded Function Dental Auxiliaries Would Benefit Consumers, Dentists and Taxpayers,* HRD-80-51, Report to the Congress (Washington, D.C.: General Accounting Office, March 7, 1980), p. 122.

Table 2. Rationale Provided by Boards of Dentistry for Prohibiting
Use of EFDAs to Complete Restorations

Restrictive States Responding to GAO Questionnaire	Rationale Provided*				
	EFDAs Lack Necessary Training	EFDAs Lack Necessary Skill and Judgment	Enough Dentists	Dentists Voted to Maintain Restrictions	Board Did Not Provide Rationale
Alaska					X
Arizona	X				
Arkansas					X
California	X		X		
Connecticut		X			
Delaware					X
District of Columbia					X
Florida		X			
Georgia		X			
Hawaii	X				
Idaho	X				
Illinois					X
Iowa					X
Kansas					X
Louisiana					X
Maine					X
Maryland					X
Massachusetts					X
Michigan	X				
Minnesota			X		
Montana					X
Nebraska					X
New Hampshire	X				
New Jersey					X
New Mexico				X	
New York		X			
North Carolina		X			
North Dakota	X				
Oregon					X
South Carolina					X
South Dakota			X		
Texas		X			
West Virginia					X
Wisconsin	X				
Total	8	6	3	1	17

Source: Comptroller General, *Increased Use of Expanded Function Dental Auxiliaries Would Benefit Consumers, Dentists and Taxpayers*, HRD-80-51, Report to the Congress (Washington, D.C.: General Accounting Office, March 7, 1980), p. 47.

*Although 17 states provided a rationale to the GAO, column totals combined equal 18 because California provided 2 reasons.

services. Thus the GAO's strategy in raising the issue is not so much informational as it is to explore the barriers with the objective of effecting a change.

A review of state dental-practice acts by the GAO showed that (as of 1977) only 10 states permitted EFDAs to perform one or more tasks associated with completing restorations. At that time, 42 state boards actually had the authority to approve expanded functions. A survey of boards revealed that their justification for restrictiveness centered on the belief that EFDAs lacked the training, skill, and judgment necessary for completing restorations. (See tables 1 and 2.) Of the nine state boards that purportedly knew of literature documenting their position, none could be persuaded to provide copies of the substantiating information to the GAO.

McBride, in a 1974 *Yale Law Journal* article, stated that:

The failure of most state licensing boards to authorize broad expanded duties for auxiliaries lies in the economic self-interests of the board members (and of dentists in general). As auxiliaries are allowed to perform higher levels of expanded functions, they become substitutes for dentists in the dental care 'production function.' They therefore begin to compete with dentists, at least to the extent that a dentist, making efficient use of several EFAs, might be able to provide services to a clientele formerly served by several solo dentists. Dental board members, who are generally well-established practitioners and well-established dental society members, threatened by possible competition from dental auxiliaries may utilize their positions of power on the board to exclude auxiliaries from the dental market by promulgating restrictive auxiliary regulations.[34]

McBride went on to recommend greater judicial activism to eliminate abuses and statutory changes to eliminate the causes of abuses.

In a similar tone, the GAO notes with frustration that many state boards seem to feel that ensuring quality care for the public is incompatible with "increasing the efficiency of the Nation's dental care system by employing EFDAs to complete restorations."[35]

Thus the GAO is led to recommend that the Federal Government work "to effect changes in State laws to permit the use of these auxiliaries to complete restorations by private dentists and public health departments that desire to do so," and "To establish policies to increase their employment in federally operated or funded dental care delivery programs to the extent possible."

EFDA survey. In support of its recommendations, the GAO reported results from a 1978 survey the agency conducted. Four hundred twenty-seven dentists in California, Georgia, Illinois, and New York were polled; 83.6 percent responded with usable questionnaires.

The survey was to determine the potential impact of changing state-practice acts to favor the use of EFDAs. The specific research questions were: (1) How many would use EFDAs to complete restorations if their state's laws were amended; (2) What benefits they believed would result from using EFDAs in this role; or (3) Why they would not employ EFDAs for completing restorations.

Of the 357 respondents, 32.8 percent indicated they "definitely or probably would employ" EFDAs if their state laws were changed. Twelve percent were undecided. Table 3 shows the perceived benefits of employing the auxiliaries. Yet another point of interest is that of 117 dentists indicating some inclination to hire EFDAs, 11.1 percent said "fees could be reduced;" a rather substantial 70.1 percent said there would be "no impact on fees."

Table 4 reveals the reasons cited for not hiring or being undecided about hiring EFDAs for 240 dentists who responded. Fully 75 percent cited the reason given in the ADA's 1975 resolution (inadequate skills and judgment); 63 percent cited doubt about patient acceptance, and 38 percent expressed concerns about additional management responsibilities.

Based on their sampling procedure, GAO researchers estimated that about eight thousand dentists in the four states would hire EFDAs if their state practice acts were modified.

In addition to its survey of private practitioners, the GAO examined all federal programs that provide dental services and several non-federal public-health clinics. Results of the inquiries indicated widespread

Table 3. Benefits Anticipated by Private Dentists From
Employing EFDAs to Complete Restorations

Potential Benefit	Respondents Rating Potential Benefit to Moderate Extent or Greater	
	Number	Percentage
Ability to service more patients	95	81
Additional time to devote to more complicated procedures	92	79
Ability to provide higher quality care	62	53
Increased net income	59	50
More free time	58	50
Other benefits	7	6

Source: Comptroller General, *Increased Use of Expanded Function Dental Auxiliaries Would Benefit Consumers, Dentists and Taxpayers*, HRD-80-51, Report to the Congress (Washington, D.C.: General Accounting Office, March 7, 1980), p. 61.

Table 4. Reasons Given by Private Dentists Concerning
Employing EFDAs to Complete Restoration

Reason	Respondents Expressing Moderate Concern or Greater	
	Number	Percentage
Belief that only a dentist has the necessary skill and judgment to do work	179	75
Belief that patients would not accept care from an auxiliary	152	63
Management and administrative functions associated with use of auxiliary(ies)	92	38
Insufficient patient load	80	33
Operative dentistry (e.g., amalgam and composite restorations) does not comprise a significant percentage of services provided	79	33
ADA opposition to delegation of these functions to auxiliaries	48	20
Inadequate physical facilities	30	13
Other	15	6

Source: Comptroller General, *Increased Use of Expanded Function Dental Auxiliaries Would Benefit Consumers, Dentists and Taxpayers*, HRD-80-51, Report to the Congress (Washington, D.C.: General Accounting Office, March 7, 1980), p. 63.

support for using EFDAs, although actual use of them was spotty.

The conclusions of the GAO report, then, are that EFDAs represent an economically viable option for labor substitution; that state practice acts should be changed (with federal encouragement, if necessary) to accommodate the use of the auxiliaries; and that a sizable federal and non-federal labor market for the auxiliaries exists, if laws could be changed. In the words of the report, increased productivity gained from using EFDAs "can help alleviate dental shortages and, to the extent dentists are willing to pass on savings realized from productivity gains, can also help contain costs," (p. i).

Undoubtedly the most important feature of the GAO report is not its analysis of the probable impact that EFDAs could have, but its acknowledgment of the resistance that marks dentistry's response to the technological innovation offered by this category of worker. Dentistry's indifference to promises of increased productivity and income was noted at least as early as 1974[36] and, more recently, D. A. Conrad has aptly identified the situation as a paradox, stating that "the organized profession is resisting change in the production function for dentistry while initial findings indicate that increased utilization of expanded [function] dental auxiliaries . . . benefits the individual dental firm."[37]

Conrad suggests that the failure to capitalize on new technology is due to the fact that "dentists as a collective resist competition among themselves and from new entrants, even though individual dentists try to provide services as efficiently as possible (and thus, at least implicitly, to 'compete' for patients)" (p. 7). Reinhardt, investigating physician productivity, made a similar observation.[38] Both of these views are compatible with the rationale developed by Evans to explain why auxiliaries are not employed as widely as might be expected: because dentists, in controlling their output, are able to maintain or optimize the profitability of the dental firm.[39]

As was noted in our discussion of denturists, dentists find it to their advantage to keep their practices moderately productive and "limited" in the sense that they compete for only a reasonable portion of the available market. Hiring EFDAs and managing a high-volume practice would upset the equilibrium and unleash competition among the remaining dentists in the community. That competition inevitably would alter demand patterns, which could squeeze out the small producer. If our original entrepreneur is not prepared to run the full gauntlet of cutthroat competition, he or she is better off to "live and let live," as Evans suggests.

OTHER OPTIONS FOR COST CONTAINMENT

The denturist movement and the exploration of the use of EFDAs represent the two major avenues by which cost-containment objectives might be met within dentistry. Two other developments also hold potential, but neither has gained sufficient strength to warrant the label of "serious contender" in the battle against labor costs.

Independent practice by dental hygienists and the deployment of indirectly supervised EFDAs are ideas that have received support from some parts of the dental community. For the most part, indirectly supervised EFDAs would come from the stock of hygienists who have had EFDA training, or they would be dental assistants with additional training. In either case, this type of EFDA would be a front-line, primary-care provider who would be extending a specific range of preventive and restorative services. (They would have more extensive training and responsibilities than were ascribed to EFDAs in the previous sections.)

Recommendations for independent hygienists or for indirectly supervised EFDAs are essentially splinter developments from the long-standing, general interest in expanded function auxiliaries. They deserve mention, although many of the previous remarks concerning denturists and EFDAs apply here as well.

While there are numerous variations on both of these ideas, a rough sketch can be drawn: "Independent practice by dental hygienists" generally means that hygienists would be legally permitted to own and manage dental-hygiene practices independent of licensed dentists. As of 1980, no state dental-practice act specifically permitted such an arrangement, although several hygienists in California have opened practices in defiance of state law. Technically, hygienists in every state are required to work under the auspices of licensed dentists who provide some level of supervision.

By and large, independent hygienists would perform services identical to those being performed in dental offices: screening, dental-health education, prevention, and prophylaxis. In other cases, the range of duties would be extended somewhat to include restorative services for children. (It should be noted that these descriptions are but summaries of arguments put forth by advocates of such practices; there are very few, if any, formal proposals being considered by state boards of dentistry.)

Arguments for the deployment of an EFDA workforce take the form of a "movement" when they are used in reference to the use of EFDAs as primary-care providers (usually for children) through the public-school system or as a way of meeting the needs of under-served areas. It is argued that EFDAs can function capably on their own, with only periodic "checks" by supervising dentists. Screening and treatment planning, as well as preventive and basic restorative services, would be provided by such personnel.

Both hygienists and EFDAs would "triage" cases; that is, they would make initial decisions on which cases to treat themselves and which should be referred to more highly trained personnel.

Historically, the idea of relatively independent auxiliaries (other than denturists) stems largely from the New Zealand dental nurse model. In New Zealand, trained dental auxiliaries work in the public-school system to provide extensive preventive and restorative services to school children. Dentists handle complicated cases and provide some oversight of the auxiliaries. The program is more than 40 years old and is highly regarded by dental researchers and administrators around the world.[40]

The New Zealand model was followed in Saskatchewan[41] (among other places), where it has also proved to be a workable approach to dental-care delivery. Where such programs have been started, both internal and external evaluations have found the auxiliaries' work to be of high quality and patient acceptance has seldom, if ever, been a problem.[42] Program administrators typically feel that major cost savings have been achieved; in many cases, care is delivered to populations which otherwise would have gone unserved.

In the United States, interest in programs of this type emerged shortly after the notion of (supervised) EFDAs became more or less credible. A number of persons advocated such programs for the U.S. Several delegations of dental educators, politicians, and researchers visited New Zealand and various other countries that were experimenting with supervised auxiliaries. Debates about the subject were held in this country and considerable controversy surrounded school-nurse advocates. Then, as the economy weakened and as dental-school enrollment climbed, discussions ceased. Since 1974, the topic has received relatively little space in either popular or scholarly publications.

This gradual demise of what was once a rather radical and widely debated idea can be attributed to a number of factors.

First, the staunchest advocates tended to be from university settings. During the late sixties and early seventies, as has been pointed out, the federal government and various private foundations were concerned about an impending dental-care crisis and about addressing the needs of underserved peoples. Through their funding programs, these agencies encouraged innovative thinking and promoted the development and implementation of projects that would solve the nation's health-care problems. Because the universities had traditionally been sources of such programs, and because they needed the research and development funds, it was understandable that the school dental nurse idea caught on and was widely advocated as a possible solution.

However, as the federal commitment to underserved areas diminished, so did university interest in innovative programs. At the same time, dental associations began pressuring universities to cut dental-school enrollments, to eliminate experimental programs and to restrict their outreach efforts. Without the carrot of program funding, dental researchers and faculty had little inclination to play the unpopular tune ("School Dental Nurse") to an audience of critical dentists.

Another factor that contributed to the decline of the school dental nurse idea is the fact that there was never organized public advocacy for such a program. Certainly no record exists of any school district requesting one. Dental associations were not about to advocate such an unwieldy auxiliary, and the universities found little incentive to do so. To my knowledge, no pilot program for school dental nurses was ever field-tested in this country. The idea thus hangs on the vine like an unpicked fruit; perhaps its time will come, but for the moment it is simply a reminder of bounty unharvested.

The matter of the independent practice of dental hygiene has an even more complicated social history. As noted, the idea seems to have emerged concurrently with the general interest in EFDAs. There also may have been an influence from medical nurse practitioners who gained their independence in the late sixties and early seventies. Like dental hygienists, nurse practitioners are predominately female, working in a professional field dominated by males. A major difference, of course, is that nursing has a much longer tradition than does dental hygiene. Nurses had gained a greater degree of independence before the emergence of nurse practitioners; the nursing profession has a much larger and politically stronger national organization (and constituency) than does dental hygiene.

Another development during the seventies was that increased numbers of dental hygienists were graduating with four-year (instead of two-year) degrees, and they undoubtedly had greater career aspirations. At the same time, the women's movement gained momentum during the seventies and encouraged women to assert themselves and live (and work) up to their potential.

Further stimulation may have come from the desire of heads of dental-hygiene programs to create innovative, effective responses to the needs of underserved populations and the problem of burgeoning health-care costs. Word of the denturist movement also may have played some role in recent developments, although its influence would be difficult to characterize.

In any event, disparate factors combined to provide encouragement to various state leaders in dental hygiene to advocate the establishment of independent practices. As noted, some hygienists have done so, in apparent violation of state laws. The actual strength of the independent dental-hygienist "movement" is difficult to determine. If American Dental Hygienists Association pronouncements on independent practice were any indication, there was no strong sentiment or sense of direction within the organization in 1981.[43]

For a short time, it appeared that something might develop in the independent hygienist movement. In the late seventies and early part of 1980, the FTC was investigating the independent practice of dental hygiene as a part of a general inquiry into dental care, but the hygiene investigation was dropped by mid-1980. Without the force of an impending FTC ruling behind them, the strongest advocates of independent dental hygiene seem to have folded their sails while waiting for fresh winds of change.

It seems unlikely that there will be any significant change in either the school dental nurse or the independent dental-hygiene "movement"

during the next five to ten years. If a sharp political change were to
occur—say an administration supportive of broad-based social welfare programs—then the advocates of school dental nursing might find
a responsive audience. Were they to see their proposals actualized, it
is likely that we would see major impacts on the dental health of
school children and on dental-care expenditures. Such a political
change seems unlikely, however.

Independent dental hygiene has an equally dim prospect. Unless
the FTC reenacts its inquiry into its "case," the chances are that the
argument for independent hygiene will fall on deaf ears. The fact of
the matter is that hygienists also lack a sympathetic audience. The
public generally has a poor understanding of what dental hygienists
do and undoubtedly does not care whether they practice independently. The only people who really care are dentists. The dentists'
position is not supportive of hygienist independence for the same
reason it is not supportive of independent denturism: independent
auxiliaries would serve to break down the monopolistic control that
the dental profession consciously or unconsciously exercises.

Dental hygienists who advocate independence have a very difficult
political battle ahead of them. They are members of a profession for
which there are abundant applicants, many graduates and many
trained, but inactive workers. The result of this is that dentists can
easily hire dental hygienists in most parts of the country. Should an
advocate of independence become too active, he or she can easily be
replaced by a more docile worker.

Denturists have two advantages that hygienists do not have. First,
dental laboratory technicians (from whose ranks most denturists
come) are highly skilled craftspeople for whom a strong demand (and
relatively short supply) exists. Denturists can thus be assured of employment while advocating independence. Second, denturists can
play to the cost concerns of senior citizens.

Hygienists, on the other hand, are not in short supply and their call
for independence does not have any emotional appeal to anyone
(though it does draw an emotional response from dentists). They are
thus advocating independence from a position of weakness.

One suspects that there are other forces at work as well. The work
life of hygienists has traditionally been much shorter than that of
dentists. Hence, most hygienists now in the work force are unlikely
to be sufficiently committed to their careers to make the capital investment required for independent practice. There may be many leaders within dental hygiene who feel strongly about the desirability of
independent practice (indeed, there would likely be cost-containment

advantages from such an arrangement), but the profession at large does not seem fully behind such a move.

In any event, political power is really the central issue. The facts of the case are these: dentists have more to gain by controlling hygienists than hygienists have to gain by breaking away; the risks of trying to break away may be greater than the promised rewards for most hygienists; there is no powerful advocacy group behind the hygienists, and there is a relatively abundant supply of hygienists available in the marketplace. While the case they argue may be valid and might bring new cost-containment possibilities to dental care, hygienists appear to be crying weakly from the wilderness. Until they can mobilize a strong support group, the independent practice of dental hygiene seems a long way off.

CONCLUSIONS

At the beginning of the chapter, we asked whether dental auxiliaries offer potential for lowering the cost of producing dental services, and, if so, are we likely to see any actual impact on costs as a result of using auxiliaries.

Clearly, twenty to thirty years of research have demonstrated that auxiliary personnel can function efficiently and effectively as substitute labor for the dentist in the performance of many common dental procedures. The potential for cost containment is there: use of auxiliaries does offer us that hope. The more problematic question centers on realization of the potential: are we likely to *see* any dramatic impact on costs?

In searching for an answer to this question, we examined the social histories of four categories of auxiliaries: denturists, supervised EFDAs, indirectly supervised EFDAs and independently practicing dental hygienists. These four groups are alternatives that are technically, although not necessarily legally, available to the dental sector.

The impact that dental auxiliaries will have over the next decade depends almost exclusively on the dental profession. We have seen that the profession is highly fraternal; that is, the members are joined closely through a strong network of organizational bonds. Dentistry's socialization processes are very effective and the profession continues to perpetuate itself with little variation from the basic mold. At the national level, this professional network is able to exercise constraints on the supply of services via its control over the production of dentists and all categories of auxiliaries. This monopolistic control over supply extends down to the level of the individual practitioner in such a way that each dentist carves out his or her share of the local market, practices in an efficient (but not too efficient) manner, and thus presents no threat to other local dental practices. The economic pie is neatly divided, with no single dentist getting too large a piece at the expense of the others.

Even though there is a purported surplus of dentists, there is no evidence of rampant competition for patients. Dental advertising, although legal, is used sparingly and has made no discernible alternative of demand patterns. Likewise, dental-insurance programs have had virtually no impact on the practice of dentistry. Similarly, dental auxiliaries have had little impact on production and costs of dental services. All of these factors *could* serve to create a more competitive dental marketplace, but they have not. Why? Because of the rigidly socialized nature of the profession and the economic control it has, which enables dentists to protect themselves by avoiding a truly competitive, free enterprise market.

With specific reference to denturists, one would suspect that this new profession will follow the model of dentistry by limiting entry to the field via restricted training programs, professional standards, etc. Denturists probably will price their product slightly below that of the dentists and, having gotten a piece of the action, settle back quietly lest they disturb the market too much. In the unlikely event that entry to the field remains open, there is the chance that sufficient numbers of denturists might be produced to force price-reducing competition among denturists themselves and between them and dentists. Even so, the denture market is but a portion of total dental expenditures and the aggregate national impact would be of limited significance.

Supervised EFDAs will likely continue to be used to a moderate degree, but the incentives to dentists to continue their small-scale, limited output practices are still too strong to offer much hope for significant cost containment through an expanded use of these auxiliaries. There is the outside chance that advertising or increased production of dentists might trigger competition and, hence, more efficient practices, but there is little reason for hope at this point.

As far as school dental nurses and independently practicing dental hygienists, one can only conclude that they are anachronisms whose time has passed (along with the War on Poverty) or pioneers whose time has not yet come. In any case, the present does not bode well for them. They lack advocates with political strength and economic power. And with the present conservative approach to social programs, advicates are unlikely to appear.

The outlook for cost containment through the expanded use of dental auxiliaries is dim. Obviously, the technology is available to allow dentistry to be practiced in a much more efficient and cost-effective manner. Cost containment could be achieved through the use of auxiliaries, but only if there were widespread changes in the way dental care is delivered. If broad public programs were enacted that were based on an auxiliary workforce, then we might see a cost-containment impact. Such programs seem highly unlikely over the next five to seven years. Equally unlikely is the possibility that the dental profession will respond to the present economic "slump" by streamlining the delivery system on its own. If anything, individual dentists seem to be digging in for a long-term battle, determined to hold tightly to their traditional, relatively inefficient but profitably monopolistic patterns of practice.

There is a glimmer of hope in the power of third-party agencies. As dental-insurance coverage increases, insurance companies and employees will be increasingly cost-conscious. From their perspective, it would be economically advantageous to use auxiliaries to the limits of the law, and, conceivably, they will take the delivery of care into their own (management) hands. Thus we may see an increase in industrially owned and managed clinics, for example, through which dental care would be delivered efficiently and less expensively than it is presently. Once such models emerge, we may then see the dental profession responding with new dental-practice patterns that use cost control, rather than market control, to increase profits. With such a trend, we may indeed realize cost-containment objectives through the use of dental auxiliaries.

Notes

1. P. J. Feldstein, "A Review of Productivity in Dentistry," in *Health Manpower and Productivity*, J. Rafferty, ed. (Lexington, Mass.: D. C. Heath and Company, 1974), pp. 107-118.

2. R. G. Kesel, "Dental Practice," in *Survey of Dentistry*, B. S. Hollingshead, ed. (Washington, D.C.: American Council on Education, 1962), pp. 95-238.

3. ADA Council on Prosthetic Services and Dental Laboratory Relations, *Denturism: An Historical Review* (Chicago: American Dental Association, March 1979).

4. *Ibid.*, p. 16.

5. ADA, Bureau of Economic and Behavioral Research, *Oregon Initiative: Results of Post-Election Research* (Chicago: American Dental Association, February 1979).

96   David O. Born

6. R. G. Evans, "Professions and the Production Function: Can Competition Policy Improve Efficiency in Licensed Professions?" paper presented to American Enterprise Institute Conference on Occupational Regulation (Revised April 1979).

7. A. K. Dolan, *A Discussion of the Impact of Possible Federal Trade Commission Actions on Occupational Licensure in Dentistry* (Seattle: University of Washington Department of Health Services, July 1979).

8. ADA, Council on Prosthetic Services and Dental Laboratory Relations, "Inter-Office Memo: Data on Ontario Denture Services" (Chicago: American Dental Association, May 23, 1980), pp. 1-2.

9. R. J. Bognore, personal communication, May 1980.

10. R. G. Evans, personal communication, July 1980.

11. B. Sellars and L. Langston, *Antitrust and Health Services: A Second Look, Government Relations Note*, Vol. IV (8) (New York: National Health Council, June 26, 1978).

12. ADA, Council on Dental Practice and the Bureau of Economic and Behavioral Research, "An Analysis of Dental Practice From 1952-1976," *J. Am. Dent. Assn.*, 100, January 1980:89-96.

13. M. Shanks, *The Innovators* (Baltimore: Penguin Books, 1967), p. 43.

14. H. Klein, "Civilian Dentistry in War-time," *J. Am Dent. Assn.* 31, 1944:648.

15. D. O. Born, "Dental Manpower Planning and Distribution: A Survey of the Literature," *Advances in Socio-Dental Research*, vol. 2, (Chicago: American Dental Association, 1975), pp. v-xxvi.

16. D. E. Skinner, et al., "Evaluation of the Expanded Function Dental Auxiliary (EFDA) Training Program," Final Report (G-85) (Silver Spring, Maryland: Applied Management Sciences, Inc., September, 1979).

17. J. Abramowitz and L. E. Berg, "A Four-Year Study of the Utilization of Dental Assistants with Expanded Functions," *J. Am. Dent. Assn.*, 87, September 1973:623-635.

18. S. Lotzkar, D. W. Johnson, and M. B. Thompson, "Experimental Program in Expanded Functions for Dental Assistants: Phase 1 Base Line and Phase 2 Training," *J. Am. Dent. Assn.*, 82, January 1971, 101-122; and S. Lotzkar, D. W. Johnson, and M. B. Thompson, "Experimental Program in Expanded Functions for Dental Assistants: Phase 3 Experiment with Dental Teams," *J. Am. Dent Assn.*, 82, May 1971:1067-1081.

19. Abramowitz, "A Four-Year Study"; W. R. Hall, *Evaluation Therapist Program.* (Washington, D.C.: U.S. Department of Health, Education and Welfare, 1975); J. Lipscomb and R. M. Scheffler, "Impact of Expanded Duty Assistants on Cost and Productivity in Dental Care Delivery," *Health Serv. Res.*, Spring 1975:14-35; M. Marcus, A. VanBarlen, A. Forsyth, and D. Bleich, "Dental Productivity: A Perspective," *Inquiry*, September 1975: 204-215; W. A. Parker, "Dental Therapy Assistant: *Cost-Performance Analysis—Final Report*, Health Care Studies Division Report No. 76-006R (Fort Sam Houston, Texas: U.S. Army Academy of Health Services, September, 1976); and G. E. Robinson and E. L. Bradley, "TEAM vs. DAU: A Study of Clinical Productivity," *Med. Care*, 12, August 1974: 693-708.

20. K. E. Kilpatrick, R. S. Mackenzie, and A. G. Delanie, "General Dentistry: A Computer Simulation," *Health Ser. Res.*, 1972:289-300. K. E. Kilpatrick and R. S. Mackenzie, "Computer Simulation Model for Manpower Research," in *Research in the Use of Expanded Function Auxiliaries*, L. Lucaccini and J. Handley, eds. (Bethesda, Maryland: USGPO, DHEW Pub. No. (HRA) 75-24, 1974), pp. 9-24; T. M. Kisko, K. E. Kilpatrick, and R. S. Mackenzie, "A Manpower Analysis of Private Practice Dentistry Thru Simulation," *Simuletter*, 9, 1978:81-92.

21. A. Reisman, H. Emmons, R. Occhionero, E. J. Green, S. Morito, S. Mehta, and T. Nunnikhoven, *Dental Practice Management: The Economics of Staffing and Scheduling*, unpublished manuscript. (Cleveland: Department of Operations Research, Case Western Reserve University, 1974); A. Reisman, E. J. Green, H. Emmons, R. Occionero, S. Mehta, S.

Morito and K. Dadachanji, *Economic and Management Considerations in the Practice of TEAM Dentistry* (Dental Clinic of North America, October 1974); and A. Reisman, H. Emmons, R. Occionero, E. J. Green, K. Dadachanji, S. Mehta, and S. Morito, "Economic Analysis in Expanded Dental Practice," Technical Memorandum No. 324 (Cleveland: Department of Operations Research, Case Western Reserve University, December 1973).

22. J. F. Blahnik, *An Investigation of Heuristic Scheduling Procedures in Dental Health Care Delivery Systems*, Master's Thesis, University of Minnesota, December 1974.

23. Lipscomb and Scheffler, "Impact of Expanded Duty Assistants."

24. Kilpatrick et al., "General Dentistry"; Blahnik, "An Investigation of Heuristic Scheduling Procedures."

25. R. Boguslaw, *The New Utopians* (Englewood Cliffs, New Jersey: Prentice-Hall).

26. Skinner, et al., "Evaluation of the Expanded Function," p. 237.

27. R. A. Hankin, "The Cost of Providing Dentistry in an Alternative Delivery Model," *J. Pub. Health Dent.*, 37(3)1977:217-223.

28. C. W. Douglass and J. M. Day, "Cost and Payment of Dental Services in the United States," *J. Dent. Educ.*, 43(7)1979:330-348.

29. P. Milgrom and D. Conrad, "Expanded Duties for Auxiliaries: Impact on Demand for and Utilization of Auxiliary Personnel." Draft Paper, Department of Community Dentistry and Health Services, University of Washington, Seattle, Washington. July 12, 1979.

30. D. O. Born, "Manpower Distribution and Costs," in *Workshop Proceedings on Current and Future Dental Roles in Primary Care* (October 9-10, 1975 and April 8-9, 1976), L. Meskin, M. Loupe and R. Micik, eds. Bureau of Health Resources Development, Health Resources Administration, Public Health Service. Division of Health Ecology, School of Dentistry, University of Minnesota, Minneapolis, Minnesota, 1976, pp. 129-141.

31. American Dental Association, *Transactions, 1975 Annual Session* (Chicago: American Dental Association), pp. 701-702.

32. Comptroller General, *Increased Use of Expanded Function Dental Auxiliaries Would Benefit Consumers, Dentists and Taxpayers*, HRD-80-51, Report to the Congress (Washington, D.C.: General Accounting Office, March 7, 1980).

33. Comptroller General, *Increased Use of Expanded Function.*

34. O. McBride, "Restrictive Licensing of Dental Paraprofessionals," *The Yale Law Journal*, 83(4)1974:806-826.

35. Comptroller General, *Increased Use of Expanded Function.*

36. D. O. Born, "Research in Expanded Duty Auxiliary Utilization: The Past and The Futures," in *Research in the Use of Expanded Function Auxiliaries*, L. Lucaccini and J. Handley, eds. (Bethesda, Md.: USGPO, DHEW Pub. No. (HRA) 75-24, 1974), pp. 85-89.

37. D. A. Conrad, "State Dental Practice Acts: Implications for Competition," paper presented at the annual meeting of the American Public Health Association. (Los Angeles: October 18, 1978), p. 14.

38. U. E. Reinhardt, *Physician Productivity and the Demand for Health Manpower* (Cambridge, Mass.: Ballinger Publications, 1975).

39. Evans, "Professions and the Productive Function."

40. R. K. Logan, "Dental Care Delivery in New Zealand," in *International Dental Care Delivery Systems*, J. I. Ingle and P. Blair, eds. (Cambridge, Mass.: Ballinger Publishing Co., 1978).

41. M. H. Lewis, "Dental Care Delivery in Saskatchewan, Canada," in *International Dental Care Delivery Systems*. J. I. Ingle and P. Blair, eds. (Cambridge, Mass.: Ballinger Publishing Co., 1978).

42. R. R. Lobene and A. Kerr, *The Forsyth Experiment* (Cambridge, Mass.: Harvard University Press, 1979); J. I. Ingle and P. Blair, *International Dental Care Delivery Systems*. (Cambridge, Mass.: Ballinger Publishing Co., 1978).

43. "Hygienists' Policy Accepts Treatment Without Supervision," *ADA News*, Jan. 5-12, 1981. pp. 1ff; "A Policy for All Seasons," *ADA News*, Jan. 5-12, 1981, p. 6.

4

Cost Containment
in Dental Education

Sheldon Rovin, Richard Scheffler, and Jeffrey C. Bauer

INTRODUCTION

Substantial discussion and analysis are being devoted to the crises be-setting professional health education. Like their counterparts in med-icine and allied health education, dental schools face many troubles and uncertainties. If these problems are not resolved soon, they could result in the closure of some dental schools or the forced or expedi-ent restructuring of programs in the schools that "survive." In this paper we advocate the necessity and desirability of planned change. The situation is analyzed from a perspective of offering constructive responses that might strengthen dental education and public confi-dence in it.

The overriding theme is cost containment. The implications of cost containment in dental education are twofold: the impact of what happens in dental schools on the cost of dental care provided to the public, and cost savings accruing to the schools because of more efficient and cost-effective academic and administrative practice. Both will be considered; the former because, arguably, much of the lack of cost-containment behavior of dentists can be traced to the role and system models they emulated in dental school, the latter because dental schools are in deep financial trouble and must find relief with-out sacrificing programs beneficial to the public.

The cost issues of dental education necessarily have many contrib-uting factors and some of the more salient are explored here. The is-sues are grouped within a framework of three basic perspectives: economics, organization and management, and education. Alternative views and recommended actions accompany much of the following analysis. The overall objective is to stimulate new thinking because so many of the current problems result from tradition and conventional wisdom no longer appropriate in a new era in higher education.

ECONOMIC ISSUES

The costs of dental education sooner or later affect applications and enrollments, practice characteristics, dental-care supply and demand, dental manpower, and other significant attributes of the dental marketplace. As is shown in the following discussion, the increasing costs of dental education can profoundly affect the practice of dentistry and, perhaps most significantly of all, the dental health of the American public.

Student Indebtedness

No cost-containment issue has more immediacy than student indebtedness. One study estimates conservatively that student indebtedness upon graduation will average $40,000 by 1985.[1] When this amount is coupled with the conservatively estimated cost of starting a traditional solo private dental practice, the debt of a person embarking upon a career in dentistry easily could exceed $100,000. According to a recent simulation study, $81,000 of indebtedness (an educational debt of $26,000 plus a practice start-up debt of $55,000) amortized over eight years at an interest rate of 12 percent would require a debt service of $16,000 per year.[2] The annual payment would be substantially higher with higher interest and shorter maturity figures.

In response to high debt burdens, new dentists are likely to seek higher gross incomes by working longer hours, increasing fees, providing more expensive services, or increasing the number of their services. In extreme cases, dentists may be forced to declare bankruptcy. The outcome of high indebtedness is likely to be a marked increase in the cost of dental care despite national efforts to control health-care costs.

Major indebtedness also would tend to limit the graduate's choice of dental-practice mode. High debt often could force a graduating student to seek a salaried position; young dentists may be concentrated disproportionately in institutional and nontraditional settings because solo practices would be beyond their financial capabilities. This outcome could conceivably reduce the flow of dental manpower to rural areas because low-debt institutional opportunities exist primarily in cities.

Admissions and Enrollment

Rising costs of entering the dental profession also affect the decision to become a dentist. Notably, applications to dental schools have decreased over the last several years to a point where the current ratio of applications to acceptances is less than two to one.[3] Demographic trends suggest no change in this gloomy situation during the next decade. In 1992, there will be 25 percent fewer eighteen-year-olds than at present.[4] In addition, current forecasts suggest a declining rate at which high school seniors will enter college.[5] Consequently, the pool of traditional applicants to dental schools (college students) will be down by no less than 25 percent! If nothing else changes, the ratio of applications to acceptances will approach one-to-one. When the demographic projections are coupled with rising tuitions that result from inflationary increases in the cost of training students, the situation could be catastrophic to schools that depend on student tuition for substantial amounts of their income. Until recently, private schools were the most vulnerable. Now, some public dental schools also are under pressure to raise tuitions to compensate for declining subsidies from state legislatures.

To the potential student, the indebtedness incurred by going to school and starting a practice will be increasingly a major deterrent to applying to school in the first place, and its impact will tend to be greatest on students from low-income groups. Ironically, at a time when the barriers to obtaining admission to dental school have finally been lowered for students from low-income racial and ethnic minorities, progress may be negated by the high cost of training and declining subsidies.

Quality of Applicants, Students, and Graduates

The decrease in the number of applicants to dental school is disturbing, but the problem is not only pecuniary. Some observers have suggested that the quality of applicants will diminish with the size of the pool of applicants. However, in the early 1960s the ratio of applications to acceptances was much less than two to one,[6] yet no one has argued that the dentists who matriculated in the early sixties are qualitatively different from their colleagues of earlier or later years. Therefore, diminution in student quality resulting from having fewer applications should not be a concern at this time.

A recent simulation study of decreased enrollment in medical schools supports this contention. It suggested that a 38 percent decrease in accepted applicants would result in a decline in quality of only 11 percent as measured by MCAT scores.[7] In dentistry, available evidence shows that the decline in applicants has not adversely affected the academic quality of the students; grade-point averages of first-year students have not dropped, and the number of students holding baccalaureate degrees has continued to climb.[8]

Although a positive correlation between number and quality of applicants has been advanced, this thesis remains untested. The qualitative criteria currently used to grant admission to dental schools hinge almost exclusively on grade-point average and the Dental Aptitude Test score. Although student rankings under these criteria generally indicate how well a student is likely to perform as a student, they are not demonstrably related to a student's eventual performance as a dentist. The otherwise bleak admissions situation could have a positive impact if it forced dental educators to focus on the meaning of the phrase "qualified applicant." Ways should be sought to identify the personal attributes (e.g., motivation, conscientiousness, concern for public welfare) that ultimately relate to the practice of high-quality dentistry.

Income (Rate of Return to Training)

The demand for dental education has been viewed by some economists as depending, in part, on the economic rate of return on the student's investment in dental training. This investment involves substantial direct costs (e.g., tuition, books, equipment, living expenses) and some equally important indirect costs in lost income. This "opportunity cost" is the income the dental student could have earned by working instead of attending dental school. The net return to an investment in dental education is based on the difference between the graduate's dental income and the income (opportunity cost) that would have been earned in the alternative, nondental career, plus the direct costs of the education. According to economic theory, the investment in dental education is rational if the extra income earned from dentistry provides a rate of return greater than that which could have been earned by pursuing the alternative investments. (See the Appendix of this chapter for a more complete explanation.)

The rate of return to training (RRT) is emphasized because applicants to dental school have been influenced by it.[9] With a lag of one or two years, applications have moved in the same direction as the apparent RRT. From 1960 to 1970, estimated RRTs rose substantially and, in some of these years, they exceeded those of medicine.[10] The number of applicants to dental school rose during the same period. Although causality is not proved by these observations, the correlation between the volume of applicants and the RRT is consistent with the predictions of economic theory.

Because published calculations of the RRT in dentistry are available only through 1970, we prepared an estimation of the RRT for a more recent year, during a period when applications declined. Using a methodology similar to that used in previously published studies, we calculated the RRT for 1977 (see table 1, option 1) to be 17 percent, a dramatic drop from 25.5 percent in 1970. This decline, coupled with the recent decline in applications, supports the hypothesized economic link between the RRT and the demand for training.

Table 1. New Estimates of the Rates of Return to Dental Training (1977)

Option	Percentage Rate of Return
1. Current dental training	17
2. Dental school shortened to 3 years	20
3. Add one year of residency (no tuition; $15,000 stipend)	16
4. Six-year dental program (working ½-time for the last 5 years)	13.5
5. Dental training for 4 years after high school (oppty. cost-H.S. education)	19

Data source on which estimates are based: Nash, et al., Economies of Scale and Productivity in Dental Practices (Research Triangle, N.C.: Research Triangle Institute, October 1978), p. 1.

Note: In table 3 of the Appendix, these estimates are compared with those based on data from the ADA. The Research Triangle data appear to be more accurate.

The RRT may also be used to compare the economic effects of proposals to ease the enrollment problem. For example, our calculations of the RRTs resulting from shortening or lengthening training are 20 percent and 13.5 percent respectively, as shown in options 2 and 4 in table 1.

Future RRTs are unpredictable, as shown by a 1980 reexamination of a 1970 statement by P. J. Feldstein: "Since it is likely that dental incomes will continue to rise in the future as a result of the many factors affecting the demand for dental care discussed earlier, higher rates of return to dental education are likely to persist, if not increase. Such increased dental incomes will, we believe, more than offset increased tuition costs and increases in foregone earnings."[11] The incorrectness of the prediction shows that projections of the RRT in dental education should be done with great caution. Finally, the RRT is only one of many considerations related to the demand for dental training;[12] it has to be weighed against social and educational factors that may be more important, e.g., the belief that qualified people have the right to seek dental training for its educational or social value irrespective of the cost of dental training or the need for dentists.

Mechanisms to Cope with Indebtedness and Enrollment Problems

One suggestion is to accept older students. No available evidence suggests that a dentist graduated at age forty or forty-five would be any less capable than one graduated at age twenty-five. Students entering dental school in their late thirties, for example, are likely to be more experienced, mature, and certain of their career goals than their younger counterparts. Also, an older person entering dental school presumably has worked elsewhere and may have the financial resources to pay for dental education without incurring the debts usually assumed by younger applicants. Of course, the RRT is probably lower for an older graduate who has fewer years to reap the return on dental education, but the significance of this fact is unknown. Indeed, older graduates who have been successful in earlier careers might be more devoted to the public-service aspects of dentistry, or they may have the business skills to operate efficient practices immediately upon graduation.

A second recommendation is to develop self-paced curricula to allow students to go to school and work concurrently, an idea that has already been tried in dental education.[13] Individualized or self-paced curricula once were used by a few schools as part of experiments with three-year curricula. Devising a self-paced curriculum (independent of the three-year objective) is easy and could provide many students an opportunity to attend school over an extended period and to earn income sufficient to keep their indebtedness low. Stretching out training may actually decrease opportunity costs and increase the RRT, depending on the extent of employment. As shown in option 4 of table 1, a half-time job and six-year education yields a relatively low rate of return, but the RRT would be higher if the student worked full-time. The night-school option that is available to law students may at least merit consideration for application in dental education. (A night school for dentistry would help resolve some other problems that are discussed elsewhere in this paper, particularly the need to provide more convenient service to patients.)

Early graduation for students who demonstrate suitable competency is a third option to counteract problems of enrollment and indebtedness. Shorter time in school was in vogue in the early 1970s, but in almost every instance the curriculum was not actually shortened; it was simply compacted into less time.[14] Like most educational innovations, it was not truly tested before it was discarded.[15] From an economic point of view, a shortened time in school obviously could have positive effects for many students by producing an increased RRT (table 1, option 2). Awarding credit for competency gained in previous studies or through work experience would be a logical component of efforts to shorten the curriculum.

Fourth, dental schools should advertise for students by pointing out the benefits of dental education, by entreating older students to apply and by extolling the advantages of their (innovative?) curricula; just as undergraduate colleges recruit athletes, so too, could dental students be recruited. Advertising in the various media is not an inappropriate mechanism for recruiting students, although it may seem repugnant to some. If the dental schools want more applicants, they will have to engage in marketing, first by discovering what potential students want and then by advertising its availability.

Dental schools might also attract more and different categories of students if they reformulated the "product" of dental education. Examples of such innovation could include the preparation of experts in dental wellness, training in the management of large-scale *private* dental-care delivery systems (a private-sector equivalent to public-health dentistry), and explicit preparation for practice in foreign countries (the "export" sector).

A fifth possibility in confronting any decline in dental education is consolidating dental schools through closing or merger. Given current trends in applications and government subsidies for higher education, school closings are no longer unthinkable. The possibility of closing or merging will be anathematic to many dental educators, but it would not be so to a conservative state legislature or to a private university having trouble making ends meet. Alternatives to closure include merging dental schools within a region and designating certain schools to be mission-specific, i.e., some schools would train only specialists and drop their doctoral (undergraduate) programs while the others would drop their specialty (graduate) programs and train only doctoral students. Getting schools to cooperate in such a venture is no mean task, and circumstances may necessitate government intervention, ranging from nationalization of dental schools to creation of a program of grants to universities that voluntarily participate in consolidations that reduce the number of dental schools.

Finally, alternative fiscal mechanisms could be developed, for example, a mechanism whereby student loans could be amortized and repaid over a much longer period of time than is possible now, like a thirty-year mortgage on a home.[16] Other approaches might include some form of national loan support as suggested in a Carnegie Commission report;[17] loan repayment restructuring (deferment of early payments or graduated repayments);[18] tax incentives tied to the provision of care to lower socioeconomic groups; a tax credit tied to the amount of income tax paid on practice earnings; guaranteed refinancing; and tuition forgiveness in exchange for future service in designated rural or urban areas, as is done in Colorado.

Higher tuitions could have a harmful effect on dental schools if they rise to a point where potential students cannot find any way to pay for dental education. At this extreme, dental schools would lose part of their revenues from tuition and fees. For 1979, total revenues from tuition fees comprised 19.2 percent of all revenues reported by dental schools. But the difference between public and private schools is noteworthy. For public dental schools, 8.6 percent of overall revenues came from tuition and fees; the corresponding figure for private schools was 37.9 percent.[19] On the surface, private schools appear to be at greater risk because they are more dependent on student revenues, but many state schools may face comparable problems as state legislatures reduce subsidies and shift a greater share of the financial burden to students. In either case, student tuition problems could aggravate revenue problems.

Supply, Demand, and Manpower

The declining RRT may be a signal that the supply of dental-care services is coming into balance with demand. The increasing number of dentists per capita also suggests this possibility. However, the situation could change significantly in the decade ahead, so careful and cautious analysis of supply and demand is indicated.

The productivity of dental manpower is a major consideration on the supply side of the market, but the factors that affect productivity are complicated. The organization of the delivery system, the method of reimbursement, and especially the utilization of dental auxiliaries all affect productivity.[20] The importance of productivity can be demonstrated by the following example. If 100,000 dentists are in active practice and some factor leads to an increase in productivity of only 2 percent per year, the equivalent of 2,000 more dentists is created—without any of the costs of training 2,000 new dentists. Since this perfectly plausible creation of 2,000 new dentist-equivalents of output equals one-third of all dental students who started school in

1980, the potential trade-off between improvements in productivity and increases in the number of dentists has obvious and striking implications.

On the demand side, a crucial consideration is the future of third-party payment. If dentistry follows the pattern of medicine, the growth trend in third-party payment is bound to rise, possibly steeply. If this occurs, then the apparent balance between supply and demand will be out of kilter and a greater supply of dentists will be needed to meet the additional demand. Likewise, more dentists may be demanded as a result of advertising by dentists or increases in public concern about dental health.

The related issues of dental manpower training can be expressed in terms of four options. Manpower can increase, decrease, stay the same, or the manpower mix can change. Professional sentiment and political considerations weigh heavily against increasing the number of dentists. Even if incontrovertible evidence were to show that more dentists would contribute to cost containment, the likelihood of this happening is slim. Few, if any, dental schools are physically capable of expanding their enrollment, and the creation of new dental schools is opposed by the government, which is the only likely source of support for such action. The machinery to increase the number of dentists precipitously simply is not in place, nor is it ever likely to be. While this circumstance presumably worries very few observers, the point is important. Today's circumstances are tenuous. The adequacy of the number of dentists today is not known with certainty, and conditions can change rapidly. If, for whatever reason, the demand for dental care were to increase suddenly and substantially, an increase in manpower would be warranted. For example, data show that approximately half the people in the United States see a dentist at least yearly.[21] If these people doubled their visitation rate, existing manpower could not handle the demand. Rapid growth in dental insurance also could create a shortage of dentists unless productivity rose substantially. The point of all this is that the country has gone from an apparent manpower shortage to an apparent surplus in a short time because of rapidly changing conditions, unperceived influences, or miscalculations. Aside from occupational myopia, nothing prevents imagining a reversal of the situation in an even shorter period of time owing to rapidly changing conditions.

The second dental-manpower option is to decrease enrollment in dental schools, an action that would make no expected contribution to cost containment and, if anything, might contribute to cost escalation, particularly if demand were to increase. However, reducing enrollment would create, institution by institution, what some would consider a salutary outcome: any appreciable decline in the number of students in a school with everything else being equal would create a more comfortable existence for the dental faculty and would perhaps contribute to an improvement in educational processes owing to smaller class sizes.

The third option is to do nothing and maintain the status quo. This option is the one most likely to be exercised by dental educators unless sufficient prodding occurs from outside. Historically, dental education has changed only when it has been compelled to do so by external forces. The chances of change occurring because of internal impetus are remote, regardless of how much it might be needed.

The fourth option is to change the mix of dental manpower through a combination of reducing specialty training, expanding the scope of work among general dentists, and placing greater emphasis on training of dental auxiliaries. Shifting the composition of manpower has obvious potential for achieving more efficient delivery of dental care, especially if the emphasis is placed on generalists and auxiliaries.[22] Overall expenditures for dental education also might be reduced by changing the manpower mix because the costs of training, theoretically, should be inversely proportional to the degree of specialization. (However, efficiencies in education and practice would not automatically lead to reductions in public expenditures for dental care. The prices and quantities of dental services are functions of several other variables.)

No one has good information about how many dental specialists are needed in the United States.[23] However, the relatively costly nature of specialty training is evident, and the generally higher charges for procedures performed by specialists is known.[24] Consequently, specialization itself can be linked to issues of cost containment; specialty care tends to be more expensive than the same care provided by generalists. The role of generalists is already expanding with respect to specialists.[25] This expansion is related to fiscal constraints, the public health effects of fluoridation, and the increasingly probable control of caries and periodontal disease by immunological and chemical means. Unquestionably, much of the routine work of specialists can be done as well by generalists.

The role of dental auxiliaries is a key factor of the issue of dental manpower (see Chapter 3). From an economic point of view, if two groups of health providers are equally capable of providing the same service, those who can provide it most economically (considering cost of training and price of labor) should do so. Just as generalists can be substituted for specialists, auxiliaries could perform many of the routine services being done by general dentists and specialists. Auxiliaries are considerably less costly to train, and their widespread usage would be indispensable in any earnest attempt to control cost.

A recent federal study predicts decreasing use of auxiliaries during the next decade.[26] The study contends that, for reasons of economy, dentists will be doing more of the work ordinarily delegated to auxiliaries. However, this prediction must be viewed cautiously, if not skeptically. For example, other recent data show that dentists are employing more auxiliaries.[27] The increased productivity associated with auxiliary labor is well documented, and patients clearly do not insist on receiving all of their service from the dentist. Dentists who have been using auxiliaries are unlikely to stop using them, so the predicted decline in use of auxiliaries is doubtful. Furthermore, a dentist's decision to perform an auxiliary's task would be uneconomic if equal or greater revenue could be generated by fewer hours of more efficient production based on appropriate delegation of work to auxiliaries; hence, dentists are likely to work smarter, not harder.

A tight economy has stimulated the practicing profession to pressure dental educators to de-emphasize auxiliary programs. If dental education responds as usual, it will accede to these pressures, particularly if the government withdraws its support for auxiliary training. This predictable outcome would be unfortunate. The best chance for cost-effective (full) use of auxiliaries in dental practice is if dental students and student auxiliaries learn to work together as a matter of course.

Manpower Planning

The need for improved manpower training is unquestioned. In contrast to the helter-skelter approach taken in the past, a reasonably planned program of dental-health manpower training must be developed now if the dental-care sector is to respond rationally to the economic turbulence certain to be encountered during the decade. A reasonable plan should have several characteristics. It should, first of all, encourage response based on regional cooperation rather than national directives. Manpower needs vary substantially across the country, and a national plan is unlikely to account for these differences. (The federal planning mechanisms of P.L. 93-641 have not been demonstrably successful in meeting objectives at a national level.) Regional solutions are also more likely to lead to innovative solutions that could be duplicated elsewhere. Furthermore, regional manpower needs are easier to assess because so many dentists practice in areas near the dental school from which they were graduated.[28] However, localized planning would require the cooperation and collaboration of at least several dental schools within a given region. Considering the difficulty in getting agreement about an issue from an entire faculty at a single school, getting faculty at several schools to agree on a plan would surely be difficult—particularly when some might be asked to relinquish cherished programs.

A second feature of a reasonable manpower plan would be to match enrollments with regional needs. Enrollment targets should be established for auxiliaries, general dentists and specialists. Targets should be predicated on regional requirements for dental personnel as determined by regional disease-prevalence rates, extent of fluoridation, supply and demand indicators and socioeconomic factors; they should not be related to dentist-to-population ratios because they have no value for planning.[29] Enrollment targets also should take into consideration regional in- and out-migration patterns. The schools in the region could then negotiate their share of the corresponding enrollment changes on a two- to three-year basis, as targets are adjusted.

A third aspect of manpower planning should be flexibility. A manpower planning system should have sufficient flexibility and adjustability to enable the proportions of specialists, general dentists, and auxiliaries to be altered as circumstances change. In the past, manpower planning has failed because it has not considered shifts in demographic, social, economic and epidemiologic conditions. Training programs should be responsive enough to gear up and down to meet external changes.

Health Care and Disease Care

The distinction between health care and disease care is important, for both health and cost reasons. Diet, personal oral hygiene, and water fluoridation are the conditions most related to dental health, i.e., the maintenance of a disease-free mouth. But dental education and dental practice are heavily concentrated on the care of disease. We have in this country an excellent dental-disease-care system, but we cannot lay claim to a good dental-health-care system. Teeth are replaced and the consequences of dental disease are repaired and palliated with consummate technical skill and costly technology, albeit for a relatively small percentage of people.[30] At the same time, dentistry does a far less laudable job in preventing dental disease and maintaining good dental health for most of the American people,[31] despite the availability of the requisite knowledge and technology.

In dental schools, disease prevention is not a school-wide concern because, although it occupies a position of importance, it remains subsidiary to the teaching of curative and reparative skills. The common lack of institutional recall systems, the mainstay of effective preventive practice, is the most telling sign of the place of prevention in the hierarchy of values in many dental schools. Dental faculty generally do a poor job of teaching disease prevention because their interests are primarily in treatment. Their reward systems, both personal and peer, depend on how well they perform as diagnosticians and technicians. The professional orientations of most dental teachers are not those that, if emulated by students, would lead to a preventive orientation.

Health-oriented dental care involves skills different from those of technical dentistry. It involves motivating and facilitating patients to learn to do certain things for themselves. Dentists are not usually trained to do this and patients do not usually expect it. This point is not trivial. The professional ethos is to maintain control: the patient must depend on the dentist. Preventive dentistry cannot achieve its full potential unless dentists relinquish control and help patients take charge of their own health.

Preventive dental skills are infinitely more difficult to teach and practice than technical skills, particularly among students who are selected on the basis of criteria unrelated to communicating and facilitative ability. There are no easy outcomes to evaluate in preventive dentistry, because health maintenance is open-ended. The problem is compounded because many dentists simply do not believe they can prevent periodontal disease,[32] and prevention entails simple procedures that command lower fees.[33] (A key challenge in today's dental education might be to develop effective financial incentives so that both dentist and patient will have sound reasons to preserve dental health.)

Much more time in dental-school curricula needs to be given to the proper training, skills, and attitudes involved in dental disease prevention. This would require faculty consent to remove something else in the curriculum to make adequate time available. It also requires that faculty members become appropriate role models. Lamentably most dental faculty members are apparently not eager to do either.

If the dental-health status of the population increases, the need for dental-disease care would decrease correspondingly. Patients with healthy mouths need less dental care and incur less cost individually and collectively. For this happy situation to obtain, however, dental education must separate health care from disease care so that suitable attention can be devoted to teaching disease prevention. Or the responsibility for prevention must be given to someone other than the dentist.

The notion of assigning to someone else the responsibility for disease prevention has also been suggested in medicine for much the same reason that the issue has been raised here: successful prevention may require a provider who is not preoccupied with the usual canons of treatment. George Silver writes that physicians should relinquish their responsibility for preventive services to preventive-service minded people; he also states that where preventive systems work best, nurses play the major role.[34]

Silver's idea has direct application to dentistry. It is attractive because a new cadre of personnel does not have to be developed: one is readily available—the hygienists. The student of dental hygiene learns more about the precepts of prevention than the dental student; most dental-hygiene faculty members come closer to modeling proper "preventive" attitudes than their counterparts in dentistry. Training hygienists to assume the role of the "preventive person" could be highly cost-effective. No additional curriculum would be needed because hygiene students are so overtrained in much of the work they are allowed to do that the time to learn the communicative and facilitative skills could easily be fitted into existing curricula.[35]

ORGANIZATION AND MANAGEMENT ISSUES

A major contributor to dental education's plight is the dated administrative organization of most dental schools and, often worse, the way they are managed. Stated succinctly, the typical organizational structure is inimical to efficient and cost-effective operation. Dental schools are organized along departmental or specialty lines. Each department is responsible for teaching its discipline to students and, generally, the departmental curriculum is not subject to review or oversight by another body or department in the school. Nominally, curriculum committees bear this responsibility, but they seldom exercise it seriously. Over the years, departments have become fiefdoms whose goals and interests often supersede or are antithetical to schoolwide goals and interests. Faculty loyalties are to departments, the wellsprings of salary raises and promotions. Multidisciplinary and schoolwide programs simply cannot overcome such rigidity. When a new program, e.g., general dentistry or auxiliary training, is manifestly needed, the system often prevents drawing on existing resources from the departments or otherwise redirecting effort. The net result is that the new program becomes an add-on, requiring additional resources and raising the cost to the school.

The prevailing organizational system is woefully inflexible. Existing departmental resources and programs are sacrosanct. Departments generally do not contribute to schoolwide programs unless they are lured by additional funding or perceived self-aggrandizement. Rarely are they compelled to do so by administrative fiat. This behavior was tolerable, even condoned, as long as external funding was available as it was until recently. But the era of government largess is over. Most new programs will have to be built at the expense of existing programs, through the reallocation of resources and the diversion of funds from one or more departments because additional funding either will not be available or, at best, will be scarce. At a time when needed most, the dynamic organizational structures and adaptive, flexible administration of resources are simply not in place. Departments are so entrenched that attempts to change them evoke fierce resistance or vilification of the administrator trying to effect the change. The existing situation, administration versus faculty, does not augur well. In the eighties, innovative cooperation may be a precondition for survival, much less growth.

Form versus Function

Dentistry evolved to carry out a function: the provision of dental-health care to society. Because it valued dental care, society sanctioned the development of an organization to carry out that function. This organization assumed the form of the profession we call dentistry. But the function (public service) has been subordinated to the form (organization) during the course of the profession's development. This distinction between form, i.e., the profession, and its fundamental function is important. Organizations are evanescent. They come and go or change, but the function remains—at least as long as society values it. A vaccine for caries or periodontal disease suddenly could render the profession as it now exists less necessary or even superfluous, but the public's need for dental-health care would remain.

As a result of the Flexner Report,[36] dental education's proclivity to emulate medical education and the major universities that emphasize graduate education led it to develop organizational structures characterized by the dominance of specialized departments. These structures have remained virtually unaltered during the past three decades, a time of great change.[37] Specialization still dominates because faculty members often confuse their primary function—training dental personnel to care for the general needs of the public—with a subsidiary function of training specialists for a relatively limited number of people. Specialization in organizational structure also endures because it represents a way of life for some faculties.

An annoying new game, characterized by such concepts as "cost containment," "cost effectiveness," and "efficiency," has arisen. Dental schools are generally trying to play the new game by old rules, but old rules no longer work. In the eighties, dental schools will have to be cost-effective. Prestigious departments or faculties with international reputations will not insure survival over the next ten years. Successful schools will make optimal use of available resources to achieve well-defined academic goals; they will have a built-in organizational capacity for change so that they can adjust to circumstances; they will have ongoing planning mechanisms geared toward programs rather than departments; and in successful schools the faculty will be committed to the overall institution, not only to a subunit of it.

Form follows function. As the schools alter their functions, as they surely will, they must likewise alter their organizational structures. Departmental interests must be subordinated to schoolwide interests if dental schools are to deal successfully with the issues likely to confront them. Departments do not have to be scrapped; they can be embodied into organizational forms that maintain their integrity but at the same time make contributions to interdisciplinary school programs. One such form will be considered next.

Management

Adaptive changes in organization must be accompanied by appropriate changes in management. Experimentation and research in management must be encouraged, the sooner the better! One widely accepted system of management, matrix organization, preserves the departments within the context of a programmatically oriented school. The matrix concept[38] involves vertical and horizontal integration of responsibility according to the program and function expected of the faculty. It requires, in some instances, dual accountability. For example, a clinical instructor might have two responsibilities: to train students in the clinic and to ensure that the clinical care provided by be accountable in the first instance to a faculty administrator such as a program director or department head, and in the second instance to a nonfaculty manager responsible for clinical care. The system requires more sophistication than is commonly found in dental-school management, but it is easily understood and implemented even by managers with little experience. Most important, the matrix system can be learned readily even without a background in management.

Attempts to introduce any kind of management system from the corporate world are likely to be met with either antipathy or suspicion.

Faculty members seldom see the need to be concerned with management, a belief now ingrained because management has been either nonexistent or unrelated to their professional life. Chief administrators, including deans, are usually regarded more as academic leaders than as principal executive officers. While they must raise money and oversee its allocation (typically by department!), general administrative and managerial skills are not required to maintain their positions.

With few exceptions, the people attempting to manage the dental schools' large patient-care enterprises are ill-equipped for the managerial aspects of their jobs. More often than not, faculty members ascend to management positions because they have excelled in teaching or research. Revered tradition dictates that dental schools and their clinics must be managed by dentists. While many make valiant efforts to succeed, most are unaware of the basic principles of management. The situation is confused. Dentists unquestionably are needed to instruct students in patient care and the resolution of patient grievances, but not to arrange schedules, purchase materials, bill, collect fees, and assign supervisory and auxiliary personnel — activities requiring personnel with backgrounds or experience in business or management.

Two aspects of management germane to dental schools merit more discussion in the context of cost containment. First, the academic and care-delivery functions should be separated so that each can be accomplished efficiently. Much of the waste, inefficiency, and general sloppiness associated with the management of dental-school clinics can be blamed on the forced combination of distinctly different tasks. The academic functions of teaching, research, and committee work require different management from delivering dental care. Delivering care in a dental-school clinic ought to be treated as an enterprise of its own, managed in ways more typical of business than academe. Consequently, all patient-care facilities and operations should be managed by people trained or experienced to do so, irrespective of whether they possess a dental degree. (Obviously, if they also have dental degrees, so much the better.) In addition to the expected containment of costs through better management, students surely would benefit from working in a well-managed clinic; their exposure to competent administration should help them when they establish their own practices.

A second consideration is the need for mechanisms to ensure that people perform efficiently according to their ability and the requirements of the particular job. Dental education is labor-intensive. Economy and quality are promoted when faculty members spend most of their time doing what they do best and minimizing time spent on what they do not do well.

Three changes would enhance the likelihood of efficiency. First, clinical educator tracks should become universal. Many clinical faculty members are first-rate teachers, but they lack either the skills or the inclination to do research. Research activities are wasteful for such teachers when their time could be spent more profitably in student instruction. Many dental faculty members feel constrained to "do research" and spend countless hours doing trivial projects in order to publish something. The dental literature is replete with the dubious results of their half-hearted efforts. Good investigation takes time. Carrying research ideas to fruition requires commitment that is not possible in light of the demands placed upon clinical teachers.

Second, part-time clinical faculty should be used much more efficiently and effectively. Practicing dentists can and should contribute to the teaching programs of dental schools. They bring to students both a glimpse of the real world to be faced after graduation and practical know-how. However, these benefits pose corresponding problems: sporadic attendance, tardiness, and less than full attention to their responsibilities at school are common. Remedying these deficiencies may not be easy. In most dental schools, part-time faculty members outnumber full-time faculty; schools often are substantially dependent on them even in basic clinical programs. Few schools have enough full-time faculty members; the situation engenders a certain vulnerability.

From a management standpoint, these circumstances are untenable. Anything less than a reliable and fully attentive teaching staff is inimical to the sound conduct of the clinical training program. In particular, part-time faculty appointments must be made with an explicit understanding of the attendant obligation. These appointments should not be made indiscriminately, and, if possible, they should be competitive and prestigious; a dentist wanting an appointment should not receive it automatically. The schools could probably do just as well with fewer part-time faculty than at present if those at hand were used more effectively. Obviously, much more leverage could be obtained if the remuneration of part-time faculty were more than token, as it is in most instances. An incentive plan of some sort, such as reimbursing part-time teachers on the basis of the productivity of their students, might help mitigate some of the problems schools are having with part-time faculty.

Third, tenure should be reexamined and, possibly, redefined. Obviously, tenure is a hazardous issue, but it is highly relevant to cost-containment objectives, particularly the efficient use of existing personnel. Every school probably has at least some teachers who have turned tenure into a sinecure: even a few of these can hurt a school that is pressed for resources. The question of incentives provides an even more important reason to reexamine tenure. Some dental schools are overtenured now, and the situation is likely to worsen. This situation weakens the incentive for junior faculty to excel. The rhetoric about the "search for truth" and other selfless goals notwithstanding, academics are motivated by incentives. If the opportunity to achieve tenure is curtailed, then other incentives must be substituted. Quality performance requires suitable rewards if it is to be sustained. Some alternative incentives might include multi-year contracts in lieu of tenure, bona fide opportunities to continue without tenure based on performance, and opportunities to be trained to assume other responsibilities or positions within the school.

EDUCATIONAL ISSUES: PATIENT CARE, CURRICULA, PUBLIC POLICY

Largely under the guise of educational requirements, patient care in dental-school clinics is inefficient, cost-ineffective, often inappropriate to patient needs, and sometimes dehumanizing. At the same time, most of the care is technically proficient, if not excellent. Patients spend unnecessary hours in dental chairs waiting with their student dentists for instructors to approve procedures or steps, many of a minor nature not truly requiring supervision. Clinic hours are almost always nine to five, strictly for the convenience of the students and faculty. Patients are not accepted for treatment unless they meet the educational needs of the student. Few patients are treated comprehensively, and inordinate time is spent unproductively. In short, the system works on behalf of providers (students and faculty), not consumers.

Few competitive enterprises could survive under these circumstances. Incredibly, dental schools have had no trouble attracting patients, until recently, for two simple reasons: the price was right, and the quality was perceived as very high because the work was supervised. Patients have tolerated inconveniences because the cost is substantially less than elsewhere. Efficiency did not matter as long as enough patients came, particularly when the inefficiency could be justified in the name of education.

Now, for several reasons, the situation is changing. The benefits of community water fluoridation are being felt. Consumers, formerly known as patients, are better informed and more demanding. The cost of treatment in dental schools is rising toward private-practice fees, and increasing dental-insurance coverage is affording consumers more choice about the care they receive and who provides it. These circumstances suggest forcefully that dental schools will have to compete aggressively for patients. If they are not successful, many schools may cease to exist owing to loss of revenues and teaching opportunities. Dental schools vary substantially in their dependence on patient-care fees, but the overall situation clearly shows that clinical revenue is important to financial viability. For all dental schools, 11.8 percent of total revenues were generated by the teaching clinics (9.3 percent for public schools and 16.2 percent for private schools).[39]

Dental schools cannot hope to compete unless they become centers of excellence where dental consumers want to go, not because the cost is low but because they obtain not only good value for their health-care dollar but also high-quality, convenient care appropriate to their needs. Although difficult, this goal can be achieved if two changes occur.

Faculty attitudes that say patient care must serve education should be replaced by attitudes that give the highest priority to operating patient-care facilities where students learn that they are there to serve people, not the other way around. Dental educators also must accept, incontrovertibly, that the quality of education is defined by the quality of patient care, not the other way around. Failing this, the schools cannot hope to continue to attract patients sufficient to conduct sound educational programs.

Second, faculty members will have to become real partners with students in providing dental care. For example, students might serve in faculty-owned institutional practices under faculty supervision to learn patient care and generate revenue for the school. This would be similar to the medical model of faculty supervision of residents who render care. The ultimate responsibility for patient care would reside with faculty members, not students, as it is in current practice; faculty income would be at least partially dependent on treatment rendered. Quality and productivity in this proposed model would be superintended by a faculty member, who would be responsible for a group of students. Each student would be assigned to gradually more difficult cases—the more advanced the student, the greater the responsibility. In addition to the training, students would acquire a stake in the enterprise by sharing in the income generated. In the existing system, dental students have no such inducement to be productive; in the proposed system, the incentive to earn while learning would help defray the direct cost of dental education and would also reduce the effective opportunity costs. This model offers incentives for both faculty and students to be more productive, efficient, and effective. It also indicates the kind of innovation that will be required to adapt dental education to the realities of the eighties.

To make this or any other new system work, full-time faculty members must make it work. Putting it another way, full-time faculty must become fully committed to their institutions, as argued recently by Rogers.[40] The outside private practice of full-time faculty and existing intramural practices both should adapt to this necessity. Allegiances divided between private practices and institutions will have to be reconciled in favor of education. Unless faculty members assume some fiduciary responsibility for their schools, the schools will have little chance of becoming centers of excellence, to say nothing (in instances) of surviving.

Marketing, advertising, and contracts with employers are other steps that many schools will have to take to attract patients and to compete with alternative dental-practice systems. Simply put, competition must become a way of life. To be more competitive, schools will have to operate their patient-care centers for the convenience and accommodation of patients. Hours of operation must include evenings and weekends. Actually, if department store dentistry ultimately proves successful, convenient hours and geographic accessibility will be key factors in its success. To compete in terms of access, dental schools will have to decentralize and move into the community. The number of types of nontraditional and off-campus sites for clinical training are almost limitless. Examples include hospitals, nursing homes, various institutional settings, mobile units, and university-owned or leased sites remote from main campuses. Although many faculty members may be initially unwilling to leave a school's campus, they may soon come to realize that the school's survival depends on it.

Obviously, the start-up costs of establishing remote training sites must be considered. The burden of these costs could be lessened if dental schools share sites within a specified region; schools within a given region could combine resources and share faculty at common sites for the training of students. The difficulty in establishing sharing arrangements between or among schools has been acknowledged, but there are tangible benefits. Even if the costs are substantial, the potential for related gains (e.g., clinic revenue, adequate teaching cases, "real world" experience for students, income for faculty, etc.) could more than justify the initial expenditures. Experiments of this type merit careful consideration and ought to be tried.

Curricula

The dental curriculum is a fundamental element in the cost-containment equation because dentists do the things they were taught to do in dental school. In dental school, a disproportionate share of time is devoted to a comparatively small number of procedures that generate a high portion of income. The same seems to be true in practice. To illustrate, a recent study of utilization of services covered by dental-insurance plans showed that the services used by the most people, 64 percent or more, generated 44.1 percent of the costs, while a limited service for 10 percent of the people represented 30.4 percent of the costs. The services used by most of the people were examinations, radiographs, prophylaxes, amalgams, and composites. The limited service consisted of crowns and bridges.[41] In Wintner's words, the educational establishment is perpetuating a costly, limited-access delivery system.[42]

Given the societal ramifications of cost containment and related issues, the utility and value of current curricula must be examined in light of public need. The typical dental curriculum does not emphasize the learning of dental-health services that are the most cost-effective for the general population. Students are taught to perform the highest quality of dentistry regardless of cost, rather than to perform the highest quality of dentistry commensurate with a reasonable cost, even though no available evidence suggests that high-cost dentistry affords better dental health.

Dental students are taught to *do* something: remove decay, fill spaces, cut pockets, etc. They do not learn very well that sometimes the best treatment is no treatment. They do not learn to watch and observe and exercise judgment; they provide treatment because they are rewarded for how well they do things and how many things they do. No matter how vehemently the instructors proclaim that their students are judged on how well they take care of patient needs overall, students cannot be graduated without completing a prescribed number of procedures. The model emulated by students is one of performing technical services—the more the better—and this behavior is carried over into practice. The implications for cost control are obvious.

Somehow, students should learn that good dental health does not mean that every carious lesion has to be restored, every missing tooth replaced, every pocket removed, and every patient seen twice yearly. Somehow, students should learn that every patient is different and that treatment decisions should be predicated on an individual's susceptibility and response to disease, the manner in which the individual maintains dental health, and whether the health benefit likely to result from the planned treatment is worth the cost.

If faculty are to teach these foundation concepts of cost containment, then curricula must include appropriate learning experiences, and students must have role models. Students learn what they practice and, thus, they must practice devising treatment plans that consider potential cost as equal to other factors. Moreover, students should be evaluated and rewarded for their ability to make cost judgments. Herein, though, resides a thorny conflict. Asking the faculty to evaluate students according to these precepts when students have always been judged primarily for their technical abilities and knowledge is asking faculty to acquire markedly different attitudes toward student assessment. To do this they must overcome the powerful inertia of custom.

Alternative Delivery System Models

Another dimension of the curricular problem is the absence of alternative delivery systems and reimbursement models for students. Virtually all students are prepared only for solo, fee-for-service dentistry. They do not learn the pros and cons of group practice, prepayment and capitation plans as remunerative alternatives, although these subjects are prominent in the context of cost containment. For reasons of cost containment and practice management, educational institutions must expose their students to various models.[43] When students learn only one technique or one point of view, they are being trained; when students learn how to choose between alternative ways or views, they are being educated. Sending students out to the real world to practice dentistry without a working familiarity with all dental-practice alternatives is akin to educational malpractice.

A no less important reason for including exposure to alternative delivery systems in curricula is that one of the alternatives might actually improve dental-care delivery and the way it is learned in schools. At the very least, expansion of this element of the curriculum will provide the impetus to examine the current system and particularly the way it is managed (mismanaged?).

Efficiency in Education

Expanding the scope of dental generalists and structuring curricula accordingly have been addressed earlier in this paper and in other publications.[44] In defining the curricular content for the "new" generalist, educators must ensure that new curricula are not old curricula under a new rubric. The temptation will be great to put into new curricula as much material as before. Academicians must remember that all they know and want students to know is not necessarily what students need to learn to take care of the basic needs of the public.

Dental education should be regarded as a continuum including predental, dental, and continuing education. Some of the ingredients in current dental-school curricula, e.g., the basic sciences, could be moved into the predental curriculum. In 1910, Flexner emphasized the university-based curriculum grounded in scientific principles as sine qua non for medical education.[45] Dental schools quickly established their curricula on the same principles. But nowhere was it carved in stone where or how the scientific principles should be learned!

At the other end of the curricular spectrum, many subjects currently offered in dental school under the aegis of specialty disciplines could just as well be learned later, after graduation, as part of this same continuum. Actually, some specialty instruction would be much more effective and efficient if given after the dentist has had some working experience and has developed to the point where the acquisition and assimilation of new technical information and skills could occur more rapidly. Some of the high-cost dental technology that requires extensive effort to teach students (and which students do not learn very well anyway) could be made available to the practicing dentist as part of continuing education.

Redundancy and superfluity must be reduced if dental curricula are to become fully efficient. A considerable savings in both faculty and student time can be extracted from existing curricula with little difficulty. Duplication exists not only between departments, but very often within departments. While some duplication can be justified, most of it cannot be defended on educational grounds.

An especially egregious example of educational inefficiency is the patient record; it is a universal problem in dental schools and in dental practice as well. Records of dental-school patients are big and cumbersome. They contain everything anyone ever wanted to know about a patient regardless of its relevance. Sometimes individual departments keep their own separate patient records. The result is an enormous duplication and waste of time spent in learning how to use the different forms and getting them approved. Some efficiency in both education and practice could be achieved if students learned a practical, multipurpose, single system of record keeping in the first place. The duplication attendant to the way students are taught record keeping is an example of the extravagance that can be ill afforded during a time of shrinking resources. It cannot be justified in the name of education.

The principal message here extends far beyond the obvious problem of dental schools' patient records. It illustrates the general duplication and resultant waste of time and effort found in dental school curricula. The reasons for it are simple: one department usually does not know what the other departments are doing; individual instructors often insist on doing things their own way, even at the risk of repetition, and, as noted earlier, the organizational structure fosters this behavior. To handle the problem of duplication, conditions must be reversed through the implementation of an organizational structure that permits teachers from different disciplines to work together, to know what each is doing, and to learn that they do not have to repeat material in the belief that another faculty person may not have done it well.

Dental Education and Public Policy

For the past decade, the public and the Congress have been expressing concern about the way the health professions have been fulfilling their public trusts. A number of legislative and judicial actions have brought upon the professions demands for greater accountability, more competition, and the development of alternative delivery systems.[46] These demands were not the wild machinations of disgruntled bureaucrats plotting against the profession. They were the legislative manifestations of a public weary of past performance, and wanting more for its health-care dollar than it was getting. The expected decline of federal funding for dental education is undoubtedly a manifestation of such public sentiments; cuts in federal support for health-sciences education are motivated by more than conservative inclinations to reduce the federal budget. Dental schools have never received as much federal money as most other health-sciences schools, but the level of such support—9.6 percent of overall total revenue for private schools and 4.7 percent for public schools— is not inconsequential.[47] (The situation for any individual school may be significantly different owing to variations in levels of participation in federal programs; fiscal problems will be correspondingly worse for schools heavily dependent on federal money.)

The issue of public concern about dental education is not imaginary. The public wants access to reasonable care at a reasonable cost, and it expects dental schools to provide the appropriate personnel. The power of the public to get what it wants can be illustrated vividly by the appearance of denturism. Denturists emerged into independent practice without the imprimatur of anyone in dentistry and without the benefits of skilled, experienced instruction that could be given by dental educators. More of the same can be expected. For example, school-based auxiliaries and dental hygienists in independent practice are not improbable. Yet, dental education seems placidly unresponsive: students are still being trained to "do things" in a costly, limited-access delivery system.[48]

This system is perpetuated principally because dental education operates within the constraints of state practice acts, dental societies, and accreditation guidelines that inhibit innovation or major departures from the existing system.[49] Dental education is unlikely to reach the nineties in a healthy state unless it transcends these constraints and uses the eighties to reform and innovate. Conflicts, real or imagined, should not deter dental education from designing a future and devising ways to achieve it. As part of the American public-university system, dental education's primary obligation is to the public that grants the university its special role in society.

Dental education has to decide whether it will attempt to shape the future or let the future shape it. If it chooses the former, it will have to recognize first that the inappropriate and costly educational approaches currently used do not meet the dental-health needs of most of the people.[50] Then, it will have to get on with the arduous business of making the needed changes.

SUMMARY OF RECOMMENDATIONS

There are many recommendations throughout the paper. Here we summarize the most important:

- Relieve student indebtedness and enrollment problems by accepting older students into dental school; increasing curricular flexibility, allowing students to work and go to school coterminously; actively recruiting students, and seeking more flexible means of borrowing and repaying.

- Change the mix of manpower, emphasizing auxiliaries and generalists, and de-emphasizing specialists.

- Regionalize manpower recruitment and training; build sharing arrangements among dental schools regionally.

- Remove the responsibility for dental-disease prevention from the dentist and give it to the hygienist.

- Change the organizational and management structure of dental schools to make them more cost-effective and efficient by employing corporate methods.

- Make more explicit the commitments of faculty to their institutions vis-à-vis their practices.

- Provide fiscal incentives for part-time faculty based on student productivity.

- Establish faculty-owned practices with students working in them as the basis for patient-care experience and faculty income; provide fiscal incentives for students based on their productivity.

- Establish patient care as the first priority of dental schools.

- Alter curricular philosophy so that students learn to perform the highest quality of dentistry commensurate with a reasonable cost rather than the highest quality of care regardless of cost.

- Build into dental curricula chances for students to experience alternative delivery systems.

- Treat curricula as part of a continuum of predental, dental, and post-doctoral training.

- Streamline curricula.

- Aim dental education at providing personnel who will give the services appropriate for the dental health needs of most of the people.

Appendix
Rate of Return to Training (RRT)

To make this concept clearer, we employ figure 1. Figure 1 shows two hypothetical age-earnings curves constructed for a single individual. Curve AEG represents what the individual's age-earnings relationship would be if the job market were entered in period 1, without the benefit of a dental degree. Curve CEF represents what the individual's age-earnings relationship would be if k time periods were devoted to obtaining a dental degree before entering the market. In this illustration, obtaining a dental degree requires going k time periods without any earnings, plus additional m-k periods earning less than that which would have been earned if the doctoral program had not been entered. After time period m, doctoral earnings surpass nondoctoral earnings, and for the remaining n−m periods the dental degree yields pecuniary benefits. In figure 2 the forgone earnings cost of the dental degree is given by area ABDCE and the benefit of the DDS is given by area EFG. Keeping in mind that the direct costs of the dental training would be sustained over time period 1 to k, we compute the rate of returns to the dentist by solving the following formula for r:

$$\sum_{j=1}^{k} \frac{C_j^t}{(1+r)^j} + \sum_{j=1}^{m} \frac{C_j^o}{(1+r)^j} = \sum_{j=m}^{n} \frac{B_j}{(1+r)^j}$$

where r is the rate of return, C^t is training cost, C^o is forgone earnings or opportunity cost, B is benefit, j denotes the time period in which the cost or benefit was incurred, and k, m, and n refer to the time periods shown in figure 1.

An early use of this concept in dentistry is attributed to W. Lee Hansen; later, it was updated by A. R. Maurizi (for sources, see table 1) and P. J. Feldstein.[51] Hansen's estimates

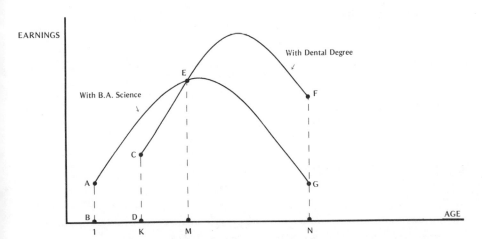

Figure 1. Age-Earnings Relationship

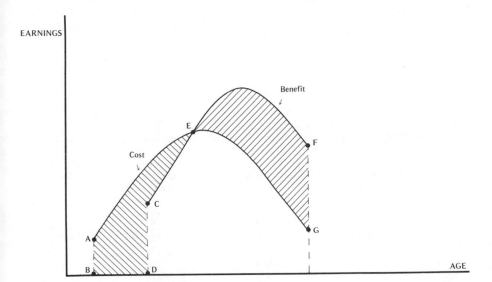

Figure 2. Age-Earnings Relationship

assume that dental training begins after high school while Maurizi assumes, as is the case today, that dental training begins after college. Are these rates high or was it profitable to train as a dentist in those years? The answer is yes, in a relative sense. For example, as is shown in table 2 the rate of return to dentistry was comparable to medicine's and in some years exceeded it.

In table 3, Maurizi shows that from 1960 to 1970 the RRT for dentists increased substantially, reaching 25.5 percent in 1970. For the same year, Feldstein calculated the rate of return

Table 2. Percentage Rates of Return to Dental and Medical Training (1939-1970)

| Year | Dental | | Medical |
	Hansen	Maurizi*	Feldman & Scheffler
1939	12.3		
1948		17.6	
1949	13.4		
1952		19.0	
1955		16.4	
1956	12.0		13.5
1958		13.6	
1961		15.3	16.6
1964		21.7	16.1
1967		21.1	18.2
1970		25.5	27.0

Sources: R. Feldman and R. Scheffler, "The Supply of Medical School Applicants and the Rate of Return to Training," *Quarterly Review of Economic and Business* 18(1), Spring 1978; W. Lee Hansen, "Shortages and Investment in Health Manpower," in *The Economics of Health and Medical Care*, Proceedings of the Conference on the Economics of Health and Medical Care, May 10, 12, 1962, The University of Michigan, Ann Arbor, Michigan, 1969, p. 86; Alex Maurizi, "Rates of Return in the Dental Profession," *Economic Essays on the Dental Profession*, The University of Iowa, Iowa City, Iowa, 1969, p. 13; Maurizi, "The Rate of Return to Dentistry and a Decision to Enter Dental School," *Journal of Human Resources* 9(4), Fall 1975.

*Zero draft probability assumption.

Table 3. Data Used to Calculate Rate of Return

Year	Dental Rate of Return	Interest Rate	Applicants (Current Year)	Pool of Eligibles* (Current Year)
1948	17.6	2.4	8,407	24,921
1952	19.0	2.7	5,178	20,121
1955	16.4	2.8	7,376	24,238
1958	13.6	3.4	6,498	30,609
1961	15.3	3.9	6,566	32.908
1964	21.7	4.2	9,988	43,220
1967	21.1	4.8	9,037	51,497
1970	25.5	6.6	11,012	57,155

Source: A. R. Maurizi, "The Rate of Return to Dentistry and a Decision to Denter Dental School," *Journal of Human Resources* 9(4), Fall 1975.

*The number of earned B.A. degrees in the physical and biological sciences for the year 1949 is the sum of earned B.A. degrees in biology, botany, zoology, geology, physics, and chemistry; for all other years, earned B.A. degrees in the biological sciences are reported as the sum of the first three fields plus other unspecified miscellaneous categories, and earned B.A. degrees in the physical sciences are reported as the sum of the latter three fields plus other unspecified categories.

Table 4. Rates of Return to Dental Training Using RTI and ADA (1977)

Option	Percentage Rate of Return	
	RTI Sample Data	ADA Data
1. Current dental training	17	15.5
2. Dental school shortened to 3 years	20	17
3. Add one year of residency (no tuition; $15,000 stipend)	16	13.5
4. Six-year dental program (working ½ time for the last 5 years)	13.5	12.5
5. Dental training for 4 years after high school (oppty. cost-H.S. education)	19	18

Sources: RTI: K. Nash, et al., *Economies of Scale and Productivity in Dental Practices* (Research Triangle, N.C.: Research Triangle Institute, October 1978) (ADA): American Dental Association, *Financial Report* (Chicago, June 30, 1978).

to be 24.5 percent without a scholarship and 26.8 percent with one. Maurizi also demonstrated that applicants to dental school are influenced by the RRT. That is, with a lag of one or two years, applications move in the same direction as the rate of return to training (table 3).

Using similar methods, we have calculated the rate of return for a year later, 1977, and our estimates are shown in table 4. There are two sets of estimates, one using data from the RTI Study[52] and the other using ADA data.[53] All of the previous studies used ADA data. The RRT for dentistry using ADA data is 15.5 percent in 1977, a dramatic decline. The figure using RTI data is 17.0 percent, also a significant drop. As predicted by economic theory, applications to dental school dropped concomitantly. In 1977, the applicant rate was about 16,500; in 1978, 14,000; in 1979, about 12,000, and in 1980, a little less than 10,000. Thus the economic link between the RRT and the demand for training is again demonstrated.

We then performed some simulations on the RRT for dental training. In option 2, table 4, we assumed that dental education is reduced to three years. As expected, the RRT increased to about 17 percent with ADA and 20 percent with RTI data. At the other extreme, we added one year of residency training, as some have suggested, to the existing four years of training and the rate of return fell 2 percent to 13.5 percent using ADA data and fell from 17 percent to 16 percent using RTI data. Turning to option 4, making dentistry a six-year program with the first year full time and the remaining five years half time as a student and employed half-time at the wage that a B.A. would earn, produces the lowest rates of all our simulations. Finally, if dental education were four years directly after high school (as assumed earlier by Hansen) the resulting rate of return would increase to 18 percent (ADA) and 19 percent (RTI).

In the RTI Study, 400 practices with about 2,000 dentists were included in a national probability sample of dental practices during 1977. Data were collected by in-person interviews and reviews of the practice files. The income data collected in this study were substantially higher than the ADA data for the same year (figure 3). For dentists between the ages of forty to forty-four, for example, the ADA reported income is about $10,000 less than that reported in the RTI Study. Although it is difficult to know which data source is more reliable, some indicators of data reliability are available. The ADA data are collected by a mail survey with a reported response rate of less than 50 percent. In surveys that ask for income data, there is reason to believe that higher income individuals are more likely not to respond. The RTI Study, by contrast, has about a 90 percent response rate and the data were collected, as noted earlier, by on-site collectors using dental-practice records. As expected, using the RTI data in the RRT calculation raises the rates. For dentistry circa 1977, the rate is 17.0 percent

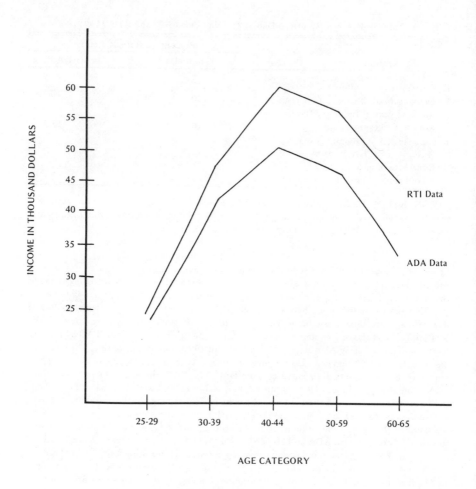

Figure 3. Mean Income by Age

compared to the 15.5 percent using ADA data. The other rates are correspondingly higher using RTI data (table 4).

These calculations confirm what many already know: the attractiveness of dentistry as a career relative to other careers has decreased. The dramatic decrease in applicants to dental school appears to correspond to the decline in RRTs. By comparison, medical education has not had a similar decline in its RRT. Although the reasons for this are complex, one important factor in keeping up the increase in medical income has been the dramatic increase in third-party payers, both public and private. In 1965, Medicare and Medicaid helped to raise physicians' incomes and today over 60 percent of physician costs are covered by third-party payers. The coverage in third-party payers for dental services has increased, but is still a very small part of the total. However, if this trend increases rapidly, as some expect, the dental RRT will rise as dental incomes increase.

Notes

1. H. L. Myers. *Proposed Loan Interest Subsidy Program for Dental Students*, a study prepared for the American Fund for Dental Health (unpublished, 1980).

2. K. Kendis, J. F. Galbally, and J. Sibner. *Identifying the Long Range Impact of High Levels of Debt for Young Practitioners. A Look at Alternative Scenarios for the Cashflow of a Dentist in the 1980's*, Higher Education Finance Research Institute, Univ. Penna., June 1980.

3. "Summary of the 1979-80 Annual Report on Dental Education," *J. Am. Dent. Assn.*, 100, June 1980:926-930.

4. R. Zemsky, S. Shaman, and M. A. Berberich. "Toward an Understanding of Collegiate Enrollments: A First Test of the Market Segment Model," *J. Educational Finance*, Summer 1980.

5. *Ibid.*

6. P. J. Feldstein. *Financing Dental Care: An Economic Analysis*. (Lexington, Mass.: Lexington Books, D. C. Heath and Co., 1973), p. 106.

7. R. Feldman and R. Scheffler. "The Supply of Medical School Applicants and the Rate of Return to Training," *Quarterly Review of Economics and Business* 18, (1), Spring 1978.

8. "Summary of 1979-80 Annual Report."

9. A. R. Maurizi. "Rate of Return to Dentistry and a Decision to Enter Dental School," *J. Human Resources* 9, (4), Fall 1975, p. 521, and Feldstein, *Financing Dental Care*, Chap. 3.

10. F. Sloan. "Demand for Higher Education: The Case of Medical School Applications," *J. Human Resources* 6, Fall 1971, p. 466; Feldstein, *Financing Dental Care*, p. 91, and Maurizi, "Rate of Return," p. 521.

11. Feldstein, *Financing Dental Care*, p. 93.

12. *Ibid.*

13. S. Rovin. "Curricular Change: Fact or Fiction?" in T. A. Smith, S. Robin, and W. H. Haley, *Individualized Instruction in a Flexible Dental Curriculum*. DHEW Publication No. (NIH) 73-437 (Washington, D.C., 1973).

14. S. Rovin. "Compaction vs. Individualization in Curricular Change," *Dental Student News — Supplement on Educational Innovation*, March 1973, p. 2.

15. "Summary of the 1979-80 Annual Report."

16. W. Kissick (George Seckel Pepper Professor of Research Medicine and Health Care Systems), personal communication. June, 1980.

17. *Progress and Problems in Medical and Dental Education: Federal Support versus Federal Control*. Report of the Carnegie Council on Policy Studies in Higher Education. (San Francisco: Jossey-Bass Publishers, 1976), p. 85.

18. K. Kendis, J. Galbally, and J. Sibner. *An Approach to the Analysis of D.O.D./State Tax Incentives for Dental Students*. Report to the Amer. Dent. Assoc. (Univ. of Pennsylvania, July 1980), p. 5.

19. American Dental Association. *Annual Report 1979/80, Dental Education*, Supplement 4, Fiscal Year Ending June 30, 1979 (Chicago, Ill.), Table 1.

20. C. Douglass and J. Day. "Cost and Payment of Dental Services in the United States," *J. Dent. Educ.* 43, 1979:330-348; J. Kushman, R. Scheffler, L. Miners, and C. Mueller. "Non-Solo Dental Practice: Incentives and Returns to Size," *J. Economics Research* 31, Fall 1978:29-39; K. Nash, et al. *Economies of Scale and Productivity in Dental Practices*. (North Carolina: Research Triangle Institute, October 1978); R. Scheffler and J. Kushman. "A Production Function for Dental Services: Estimations and Economic Implications," *Southern Economic J.* 44, (1), July 1976:25-35; J. Lipscomb and R. Scheffler. "Impact of

Expanded Duty Assistants on Cost and Productivity in Dental Care Delivery," *Health Services Research* 10, Spring 1975:14-35; "An Analysis of Dental Practice from 1952 to 1976," *J. Am. Dent. Assn.* 100, January 1980:89-96; R. Scheffler and L. Rossiter. "Methods of Compensating Dentists and Hours Worked," presented at the Western Economic Association Meeting, San Diego, June 1980.

21. *Dental Manpower Fact Book*, Manpower Analysis Branch, Division of Dentistry, HEW, HRA, BHM. (Washington, D.C., 1979).

22. J. Newman, W. Elliott, J. Gibbs, and H. Gift. "Attempts to Control Health Care Costs: The United States Experience," *Soc. Sci. and Med.* 13A, 1979: 529-540.

23. S. Rovin. "The Future of Dental Specialization: Policy Issues," *J. Dent. Educ.* 43, 1979:537-543.

24. Scheffler and Rossiter, *Methods of Compensating.*

25. HEW. *Forecasts of Employment in the Dental Sector to 1995.* Publication No. (HRA) 79-6 (Washington, D.C., September 1979).

26. *Ibid.*

27. Nash, et al., *Economies of Scale*, and "An Analysis of Dental Practice,."

28. *Dental Manpower Fact Book.*

29. Rovin, "The Future of Dental Specialization."

30. J. Newman and O. Anderson. *Patterns of Dental Service Utilization in the United States: A Nationwide Survey*, Research Series 30. (Chicago: Center for Health Administration Studies, Univ. Chicago, 1972), p. 18.

31. HEW. *Basic Data on Dental Examination Findings of Persons 1-74 Years. U.S. 1971-1974.* Office of Health Research, Statistics, and Technology, NCHS DHEW Publication No. (PHS) 79-1662 (Washington, D.C., 1979), p. 4.

32. L. Meskin and S. Rovin. "Do We Tell the Truth about the Prevention of Periodontal Disease?" *J. Prev. Dent.* 5, (4), July-August 1978.

33. George Silver. *Child Health/America's Future* (Germantown, MD: Aspen Pub., 1978); D. Malvitz and S. Judge. "Employment Patterns of Dental Hygienists in Michigan," *Dent. Hyg.* 50, 1976:463-468.

34. Meskin, "Do We Tell the Truth?"

35. A counter economic argument is related to the length of time hygienists stay in the work force. Popular opinion is that it is not very long and, thus, there would be a low rate of return attendant to their training. But there is a lot of mythology here and the only report we have come across avers otherwise. A survey of 125 hygienists in Michigan shows that 65 percent still practice an average of 24 hours per week, 30 years after their training (Malvitz, p. 41). This is higher than the 60 percent figure shown by Labor Participation Rate data for nurses.

36. A. Flexner. *Medical Education in the U.S. and Canada*, Carnegie Fund for the Advancement of Teaching, Bulletin No. 4, 1910.

37. A. Toffler. *Future Shock* (New York: Random House, 1970).

38. S. Davis and P. Larence. *Matrix* (Reading, Mass.: Addison-Wesley, 1977).

39. American Dental Association. *Annual Report 1979-80*, Table 1.

40. D. Rogers. "On Preparing Academic Health Centers for the Very Different 1980's," *J. Dent. Educ.* 44, June 1980:301-308.

41. H. Bailit et al. "Controlling the Cost of Dental Care," *Am. J. Pub. Health* 69, July 1979:699-703.

42. A. Wintner et al. "Goals, Objectives and Outcomes: Case Study of a Program Assessment," *J. Dent. Educ.* 44, August 1980:484-490.

43. R. Fein. "Health Manpower: Some Economic Considerations," *J. Dent. Educ.* 40, 1976:650-654.

44. Rovin, "The Future of Dental Specialization."

45. Malvitz, "Employment Patterns."

46. Rovin, "The Future of Dental Specialization."

47. American Dental Association. *Annual Report 1979/80*, Table 1.

48. Bailit, "Controlling the Cost."

49. *Ibid*.

50. *Report of the Special Higher Education Committee to Critique the 1976 Dental Curriculum Study*. (Battle Creek, MI: W. K. Kellogg Foundation, 1979).

51. Feldstein, *Financing Dental Care*.

52. Nash, et al., *Economies of Scale*.

53. American Dental Association. *Financial Report* (Chicago, June 30, 1978).

5

Prevention of Oral Disease

Brian A. Burt and Kenneth E. Warner

INTRODUCTION

In recent years it has become widely accepted that prevention might be used not only to improve health, but also to contain the costs of health care. The basic idea is a simple one: relatively low-cost investments in disease prevention and health promotion will prevent or postpone illness and disability that require more expensive medical care. Thus, prevention "works" as a cost-containment device if the dollars saved in future years, discounted to their present value (see section below on discounting), exceed the current cost of making the effort. It should be emphasized, however, that prevention can work as a health-care practice and simultaneously fail as a cost-containment strategy. This will happen if the health-care procedure prevents or postpones illness to the satisfaction of the provider and patient at a cost that exceeds the likely savings later.

At the outset, we wish to emphasize that the "more-is-better" philosophy, conventional wisdom for some persons, frequently does not translate into effective cost-containment strategy. Figure 1 illustrates this point by depicting the relationship between costs and benefits that result from some preventive procedures; it suggests that costs rise at an increasing rate while benefits rise at a decreasing rate. Another way of saying this is that marginal costs are rising while marginal benefits are falling. Thus, at a level of preventive activity in excess of F (figure 1), costs actually exceed benefits. Maximum net benefit, or the largest excess of benefits over costs, is attained at E (figure 1). From a cost-containment standpoint, this is the optimum

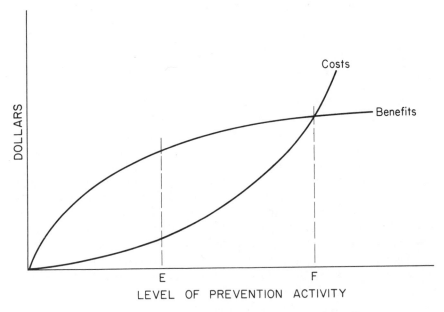

Figure 1. Hypothetical Relationship Between Costs and Benefits
in Prevention Activities

level of prevention activity. In practice, of course, it is very difficult
to determine this point of optimality, but this theoretical character-
ization serves to emphasize that the cost-containment potential of
disease prevention is rarely independent of the degree to which the
activity is pursued.

Structure of This Chapter

In this chapter, we began by introducing some concepts regarding
prevention. Our main purpose is to present an exercise in cost analysis,
in which we simulate seven "cost streams" of lifetime dental histories.
A cost stream is defined as a sequence of annual expenditures for
dental care over the lifetime (here six to seventy-nine years) of a
hypothetical individual. These cost streams, necessarily simplified,
are essentially simulated treatment histories for seven hypothetical
individuals, assuming various combinations of preventive procedures,
treatment received, and oral-health outcomes. These outcomes range
from early loss of all teeth to almost complete retention of teeth.
Existing data were used where possible to develop the treatment
histories, but a number of assumptions were required. Costs of the

lifetime dental treatment in each case can then be compared and related to the resulting dental outcomes. We have deliberately avoided characterizing outcomes as "best" or "worst" in oral-health terms, though of course we have our views just as readers will. The point of this exercise is that readers must themselves relate each outcome to the cost of achieving it.

Direct expenditures for dental care do not constitute the only costs of care. Receipt of services also involves a time cost to the patient—time must be sacrificed from other productive activities, such as work and school—and there are myriad other costs as well, some tangible (e.g., the energy costs of transportation to and from the dentist's office) and some intangible (e.g., the fear generated by contemplating or experiencing a dental visit). A conceptually complete analysis of the costs of dental care would include all such costs, imputing values to those costs for which market values are not readily available. While we endorse the inclusion of such costs in future research, we have excluded them in this exploratory analysis, principally because of the difficulty in imputing dollar values to the intangibles. While an analysis limited to direct expenditures must necessarily be viewed as incomplete, the lack of suitable empirical data demanded that many assumptions be made even in the assessment of direct costs. The exposition is more straightforward as a result of restricting the cost streams to direct expenditures, and we believe that this approach is appropriate for an introductory analysis. Ours may not be a comprehensive social-cost analysis, but we hope that it will explain the analytical principle effectively, capture costs of present policy interest, and encourage future research along similar methodological lines.

Just as costs are varied in kind, benefits range from the economically tangible—such as direct, future cost savings attributable to current care—to the intangible, including what may be the greatest benefit of dental care: the utility of having sound teeth and good oral health. In this analysis, as stated, we have chosen not to attack this conceptually and empirically difficult issue. Neverthelss, it is imperative to recognize that the consumer's perception of the value of good oral health is what drives demand for dental care, and this perception probably varies from one socioeconomic class to another. This is a theme that we would encourage other researchers to incorporate in future attempts to evaluate the relative costs and benefits of alternative streams of care.

In this analysis we have chosen not to take a standard outcome, such as preventing any loss of teeth throughout life, and seek what may be the least expensive way of achieving that goal. This decision was made because such outcomes are not often seen in real life, and because a professionally determined standard outcome may be unrealistically high. In terms of methods, it would then be virtually impossible to assess the cost of bringing public awareness of the desirability of dental health to the point where this outcome could be achieved. The variable-expenditure and variable-outcome model we have chosen means that value judgments are still required to determine what the "best bet" for prevention might be.

We have also chosen not to compare relative costs of prevention and restoration. We made this decision in part because such an exercise would be heavily caries-oriented and therefore concentrated at the younger end of life, and in part because the long-term benefits of many caries-prevention procedures are still uncertain (as will be discussed below). The subject has been examined before,[1] at least over the short term, and the conclusion reached that prevention is less expensive when the caries-susceptibility of the target population (or individual) is reasonably high. When it is not, the marginal costs of the prevention might exceed the marginal benefits. In other words, where caries-susceptibility is low, the patient pays for prevention of disease that may not have occurred anyway.

The scope of this chapter does not allow a full examination of all preventive procedures. We therefore had to make choices on what procedures to examine, guided by the evidence in the literature regarding the most effective procedures currently available. The cost-analysis exercise is therefore preceded by short reviews of procedures for prevention of dental caries and periodontal disease in which the rationale for selection of chosen procedures is presented.

Because the concept of discounting is important in any long-term economic analysis, there is a description of discounting before the cost analysis. We also include discussions of what we mean by cost-containment and prevention.

WHAT IS COST CONTAINMENT?

To date, efforts to control the spiraling costs of health care have emphasized restraints on the direct expenditures for an established pattern of health-care services, principally by discouraging "unnecessary" or marginally useful services. The centerpiece of legislative jousting in 1979-1980 was containment of hospital costs, the most visible source of medical cost inflation. Political efforts of this kind typify the general perception of cost containment as a short-term issue. Many, however, would prefer to view cost containment in the context of the maintenance of an acceptable degree of public and individual health at a reasonably stable level of expenditures over the long term. In dental care, cost containment usually is perceived by the public as restriction of direct expenditures for dental treatment, with the implicit assumption that quality of care will remain unchanged. The dental profession, on the other hand, tends to view cost containment as a double-barrelled threat that might both restrain fees and force the provision of unacceptably low-quality dental care.

A broader, long-term view of the issue, however, would require defining cost containment as the most reasonable minimization of all costs associated with dental care, including those costs associated with a failure to receive needed dental care. This concept would then comprise not only control of the direct expenditures on dental care, but also control of the indirect costs such as time required for treatment, the personal and social costs (i.e., time lost from work or school) of dental neglect, and other aspects of the loss of quality of life brought about by dental disease.

This broader philosophy of cost containment is one to which we subscribe, though as noted above, our formal analysis does not incorporate all indirect costs and benefits. We do make attempts to relate the level of direct expenditures on dental treatment to both the expenditures on prevention and the level of dental-health outcome. The implications for prevention in cost containment are that the level of dental status outcome desired is likely to be fairly closely related to the cost of the preventive effort.

WHAT IS PREVENTION?

A great deal of preventive dentistry is being practiced in the United States. Surveys from the American Dental Association (ADA) showed that over half of all practitioners prescribe fluoride supplements[2] and that almost all practicing dentists use topical fluorides in their practices.[3] In addition, 60 to 80 percent of pediatricians and family practitioners have reported that they prescribe fluoride supplements for children.[4] The ADA also reports that the numbers of practicing dentists who employ hygienists is increasing steadily; 45 percent of all dentists reported employing hygienists in 1976.[5] At the community level, half of the U.S. population is receiving fluoridated water,[6] some ten million children are regularly using self-applied fluorides in school-based programs,[7] and over 90 percent of dentifrices now used contain fluoride. Fluoride solutions for rinsing at home are now available without prescriptions in drugstores and supermarkets, although it is not known to what extent they are being used. ADA surveys also showed that the number of preventive procedures carried out by practicing dentists is continuing to increase and has increased considerably since the late 1950s.[8] All of this activity has come to be seen by many as a "prevention boom."

It is well to pause here and remind ourselves just what we mean when we use the expression "prevention." A number of preventive procedures in dentistry, perhaps all of them, need to be repeated consistently for their benefits to be maintained. Use of the procedures sporadically will have only limited benefits, while consistent use of the procedures for short periods only may merely postpone the onset of disease. In the ecology of dental disease there is as yet no analogue to the "one-shot" preventive effects of immunization for infectious diseases.

Figure 2 represents the differences between true prevention and delay of dental caries, a model adapted from a concept suggested by Jackson.[9] The line NH in the diagram represents the natural history of the carious attack, showing how it increases at a sharp rate in the earlier years of life and then increases at a much slower

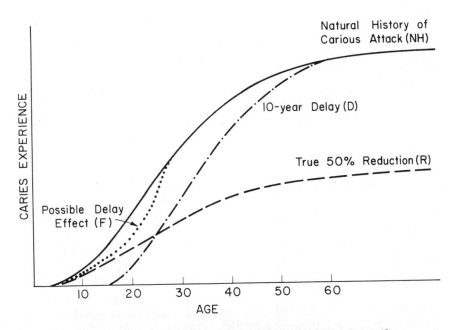

Figure 2. Four Representations of Carious Experience Throughout Life; the Natural History and Three Modifications

rate in later years. If true preventive action takes place, such as occurs with water fluoridation, then the line follows the pattern represented by line R, that of true reduction. If a preventive procedure succeeds only in delaying the onset of caries, the curve of occurrence of the disease follows line D, in this case representing approximately a ten-year delay. While we do not know the time extension of benefits resulting from a three-year fluoride mouthrinse program for a child aged eleven to fourteen, it is possible that it approximates the dotted line F. What we are hypothesizing here is that the effect of the fluoride program is sufficient to reduce the incidence of caries by approximately 30 percent, and then for several years after cessation of the program the benefits continue. But sometime in later life the line F joins in with line NH so that the lifetime caries experience has not in fact been changed. The limited evidence available suggests that some preventive benefits are retained up to five years after the cessation of topical fluoride treatments,[10] but lifetime benefits are still unknown.

If either caries or periodontal disease takes hold in an individual, the end result without intervention is tooth loss and subsequent expensive treatment to minimize further tooth loss and maintain the health of existing teeth. Therefore, no matter how effective any one procedure or set of procedures may be with respect to preventing caries (and many were identified at The University of Michigan Workshop in 1978)[11] they will be of limited value over a lifetime if periodontal disease flourishes. Similarly, an effective method of preventing periodontal disease will obviously be of limited potential if the teeth have already been ravaged by caries. The only way that prevention is going to be effective over a lifetime is if the two major oral conditions, caries and periodontal disease, are both substantially prevented.

PREVENTIVE PROCEDURES: DENTAL CARIES

Water fluoridation is dentistry's greatest contribution to public health. At the community level, there is abundant evidence to show that fluoridation reduces the prevalence and incidence of caries more than any other preventive measure.[12] It is generally accepted as the most cost-effective preventive measure in dentistry.[13] It is also a socially equitable form of prevention in that receipt of its benefits is not dependent on income, education, or access to dental treatment. At least six analyses have indicated that the benefits of fluoridation far outweigh the costs for children and young adults.[14] While there is little doubt that fluoridation reduces the cost of dental care for children,[15] the lifetime impact of fluoridation on containing costs of all dental treatment is less clear. Some reasonable estimates from limited data, however, can be made.

Jackson, Murray, and Fairpo[16] estimated that over a lifetime fluoridation reduced the prevalence of caries by 44 percent. Evidence that benefits of fluoridation received in childhood do last into adult years is shown in table 1. While the data in table 1 are not directly comparable, the considerable differences in results are all in the same direction. The notable difference in degree of tooth loss between the Aurora-Rockford[17] and the Colorado Springs-Boulder[18] studies is dificult to explain; it could be the result of a small sample size in Boulder. Murray's data from the Hartlepool-York study[19] in England are interesting; Hartlepool's socioeconomic status is lower than York's and it has a much lower dentist-to-population ratio. It can be seen in table 1 that up to age thirty-four, about the age limit at which total tooth loss could be attributable almost entirely to caries, there are eight times fewer edentulous (toothless) persons in Hartlepool than in York. Over age thirty-five, however, the proportions of edentulous persons are

Table 1. The Effect of Water Fluoridation on Tooth Loss in Adults Age 40 or Older

Community	Fluoride (ppm)	Proportion Edentulous	Mean Tooth Loss*
Aurora	1.2	2% over 20	2.69 in 40-49 y-o
			3.14 in 50-59 y-o
Rockford	0.1	14% over 20	3.65 in 40-49 y-o
			4.66 in 50-59 y-o
Colorado Springs	2.5	not stated	3.1 in 40-44 y-o
Boulder	"negligible"	not stated	12.1 in 40-44 y-o
Hartlepool	1.8	0.4% for 15-34 y-o	6.9 in 40-65 y-o
		32.3% for 35-65 y-o	
York	0.2	3.2% for 15-34 y-o	9.7 in 40-65 y-o
		35.8% for 35-65 y-o	

Sources: Aurora-Rockford: H. R. Englander and D. A.Wallace, "Effects of Naturally Fluoridated Water on Dental Caries in Adults," *Public Health Reports* 77(10), pp. 887-93, 1962; *Colorado Springs-Boulder:* A. L. Russell and Elias Elvove, "Domestic Water and Dental Caries VII: A Study of the Fluoride-Dental Caries Relationship in an Adult Population," *Public Health Reports* 66(9), pp. 1389-1401, 1951; *Hartlepool-York:* J. J. Murray, "Adult Dental Health in Fluoride and Non-Fluoride Areas: Part 1 — Mean DMF Values by Age," *British Dental Journal* 131(9), pp. 391-95, 1971; "Adult Dental Health in Fluoride and Non-Fluoride Areas: Part 3 — Tooth Mortality by Age," *British Dental Journal* 131(11), pp. 487-92, 1971.

*Dentate adults only. The Aurora/Rockford study excluded all adults with fewer than 10 teeth.

almost the same, presumably reflecting the universal impact of periodontal disease and the inability of fluoridation to reduce its prevalence.[20]

Few other data on the efficacy of fluoridation in adulthood are
available; there appear to be none at all on cost-effectiveness of fluoridation in adulthood and whether fluoridation reduces or increases
the cost of care of adults over forty. The data in table 1 seem to
indicate that adults who have benefitted from fluoridation progress
into later life with between one and nine more teeth than do adults
deprived of fluoridation. This fact of oral health could result in
either of two opposing outcomes for cost containment. These
are:

- Savings demonstrated in youth continue into later years. Not
  only do these adults have more teeth, they also have fewer
  carious lesions needing treatment in their remaining teeth.
  There are fewer restorations to require replacement and possible
  endodontic treatment. In addition, Stamm and Banting[21] have
  shown that adults in fluoridated areas have less root caries
  than in nonfluoridated areas.

- Full clearance and dentures, when assessed over time, are the
  cheapest form of treatment (in direct expenditures) because individuals receiving this form of treatment effectively drop out
  of the dental-care system. In fluoridated areas there are more
  people with more teeth who will demand more dental care to
  have old restorations replaced, periodontal treatment, or
  chrome-cobalt partial dentures or fixed bridgework. (They
  might even demand orthodontic care if they act on the advertisements that they read.) Many will still eventually receive full dentures, thereby incurring a series of expensive
  treatments.

Which of these possible outcomes is nearer the truth, or to what
degree a mixture of the two is the most likely outcome, is unknown.
The impact of fluoridation on the costs of dental care, as previously
stated, is being examined in this chapter.

In addition to water fluoridation, numerous other methods of using
fluoride have been demonstrated to reduce the incidence of caries in
children, at least to some extent. Efforts to simulate the benefits of
water fluoridation by fluoride ingestion have taken several forms.
The addition of fluoride to school water supplies in the United States
at a concentration of 4.5 parts per million (ppm) have led to reductions in caries incidence among children in the range of 40 percent.[22] The addition of fluoride to table salt in several countries has

lead to reductions in caries incidence of 25 percent in the communities where this salt is available.[23] Fluoride tablets, when taken consistently, can reduce caries incidence 20 to 40 percent in young children who have been taking the tablets for periods of two to six years.[24] School fluoridation and the use of fluoride tablets have become established public-health procedures in the United States; the use of fluoride tablets is widely practiced as a public-health measure in many European countries, and salt fluoridation is considered the most promising method of providing the benefits of fluoride to populations in developing countries.

The use of fluoride topically also reduces caries incidence. Several different fluoride-containing materials applied by dental professional personnel have all been shown to reduce caries incidence in children by 30 to 35 percent.[25] The professionally applied topical fluoride most in use today is probably the gel form of acidulated phosphate fluoride (APF); its application to children's teeth has become a standard part of dental practice. Rinsing with fluoride-containing solutions has been shown to be effective and cost-effective[26] and is used as a public-health measure reaching several million schoolchildren in the United States.[27] Research attention at the present time is being devoted to the combined uses of fluoride to reduce the prevalence of caries even further. In Nelson County, Virginia, the combined use of a daily 1.0 milligram sodium fluoride tablet, a weekly rinse with a 0.2 percent sodium fluoride solution, and provision of a toothbrush plus a fluoridated toothpaste for home use has reduced the incidence of caries in a rural population by some 35 percent after four years.[28] Further reductions in caries incidence on the order of 30 percent are also reported from the topical use of fluoride in already fluoridated areas.[29] Somewhat smaller though consistently reported percentage reductions result from the use of fluoride-containing dentifrices alone.[30]

Some lasting effects of topical fluorides[31] and of fluoride tablets[32] have been found, but it is still uncertain what the long-term effects really are. It is not known whether such uses of fluoride alter the natural history of caries according to curves R, D, or F (figure 2). Without better knowledge of long-term benefits, only limited conclusions can be reached about the lifetime cost-containment potential of alternative uses of fluoride, though most are more or less cost-effective in the short-term.[33]

Other methods of reducing the incidence of caries, such as by dietary restriction and the use of fissure sealants, are even more uncertain with respect to their long-term benefits. Accordingly we will not be considering them directly here.

From this brief examination of methods available for the prevention of caries, we decided to examine in detail only the impact of water fluoridation. Principally, this was because it has previously been judged as the most effective and cost-effective measure available,[34] and because it is the only current measure for which a reasonable assessment of lifetime benefit can be made.

PREVENTIVE PROCEDURES: PERIODONTAL DISEASE

In studies on the natural history of periodontal disease, Loe and his co-workers[35] have shown that in patients where a high degree of oral hygiene is maintained, the development of periodontal disease is practically halted. In another group in which oral hygiene was poorer, the disease progresses inexorably over time. This evidence further confirms what is generally accepted, namely that dental plaque is so strongly associated with periodontal disease that the relationship is one of cause and effect.[36] The rational approach to prevention of periodontal disease is therefore to reduce plaque levels to a minimum. While there is virtual unanimity on this principle, it is less clear just what are the best methods of plaque removal to promote in practice. Sheiham, in his review, asserts that individual motivation leading to the adoption of long-term oral-hygiene practices by the individual is the principal method by which periodontal health can be maintained. While few would disagree with this philosophy, the problem at present is that there is little knowledge on how best to achieve this goal.

Plaque removal by dentists or operating auxiliaries; at intervals of from two weeks to two months in children and two months to three months in adults, produced impressive results in Swedish children[37] and adults.[38] The plaque-removal sessions were accompanied by intensive instruction in personal oral-hygiene practices and involvement of parents and schoolteachers. Application of the same principles has been effective, both following limited surgery and without surgery, in adults in Sweden[39] and in the United States.[40] These and other studies have also demonstrated that heroic surgery is of little benefit in treating established disease and that existing antimicrobial solutions have some efficacy in postoperative treatment[41] but are of little use in prevention. Antimicrobials in the future may play a greater role in the prevention of periodontal disease, but further development is required.

The expression, "professional cleaning," now has a specific meaning in periodontal therapy. Taken from the regimen for children described by Axelsson and Lindhe in 1974,[42] it is defined as follows:

- Detailed initial explanations of oral-disease etiology (causes) and purpose of treatment by the dentist or auxiliary carrying out the treatment.

- Identification of plaque in the patients' mouth by a disclosing tablet; demonstration of tooth-brushing technique in removing the stain. Patient use of dental floss under supervision. Repetition of oral-hygiene instructions throughout the course of treatment if necessary.

- Rubber-cup cleaning of accessible surfaces; engine-mounted pointed-bristle cleaning of occlusal surfaces with a fluoride-containing prophylactic paste.

- Interdental cleaning, again by dentist or auxiliary, with dental floss and reciprocating interproximal tips.

Adults with established disease may also require root planing, curettage, and recontouring of existing restorations.

The results of these studies indicate that the most potentially effective approach to long-term prevention of periodontal disease at present is likely to be the right combination of patient education and professional plaque removal at appropriate intervals.

DISCOUNTING

The costs and benefits of prevention programs generally accrue over time, rather than all at once, and accrual patterns differ for costs and benefits. For example, the costs of school fluoride mouthrinse programs are incurred during several years of childhood, but the benefits of the program are spread over many years. How are these costs and benefits to be compared? Even if we control for (or eliminate) inflation, is a dollar today the same to us as a dollar twenty years from now? The answer is no; most people tend to value a dollar today more than a dollar next year, or ten or twenty years from now. In part, this reflects the fact that current possession of the money implies more options: one can spend the money today, or save it if one wishes to have it in the future. By contrast, receiving the money twenty years from now precludes the possibility of using it now or any time before twenty years have passed. Furthermore, saving money today implies the opportunity to invest it in productive uses which, in times of economic growth, translates into increasing its value. That is, if a dollar invested today yields 5 percent productivity per year, in twenty years the dollar will have grown to $2.65. In short, deferring consumption and investing instead in productive activity permits the value of a resource to grow over time. Thus, in this example, the *equivalent* of a dollar today in twenty years' time is $2.65.

To make present and future dollars commensurate, economists employ *discounting*. Future costs and benefits are divided by a discount factor which converts them into their *present value*. The size of the discount factor is a function of the amount of time that will elapse before realization of the cost or benefit in question. By discounting all future costs and benefits to their present values, analysts can add all costs together, and similarly all benefits, to determine the *present discounted value* of the streams of costs and benefits. To use the previous example, if the discount rate is 5 percent per year, the present value of $2.65 realized twenty years from now is $1.00 [$2.65/(1.05)^{20}]. Alternatively, the present value of a dollar twenty years from now is only $0.38 [$1.00/(1.05)^{20}]. Clearly a dollar today is preferable to a dollar tomorrow.

Discounting permits us to make sense of complex patterns of costs and benefits. It allows cost-benefit analysis — comparing the advantages of a program (its benefits) with its drawbacks (costs) to help in deciding whether the program is desirable. In addition, discounting allows cost-effectiveness analysis — comparing the relative costs of different programs that produce comparable (though nonmonetized) benefits so that we can assess their relative desirability.

To illustrate the effect of discounting on dental-disease prevention, consider a greatly simplified hypothetical example, summarized in table 2. Suppose that dental-care policymakers are contemplating recommending one or both of two dental-prevention programs. Program 1 costs $1,000,000 this year and promises to save $1,250,000 next year (e.g., by immediately, but only temporarily preventing decay). Program 2 costs $1,000,000 this year and promises to yield savings in dental-care costs of $2,000,000 twenty years from now.

Table 2. Hypothetical Benefits of Discounting on Valuations of Two
Dental-Disease Prevention Problems

	Program 1	Program 2
Initial cost ($)	1,000,000	1,000,000
Benefit undiscounted ($)		
Year 1	1,250,000	0
Year 20	0	2,000,000
Benefit discounted at 5% per year ($)		
Year 1	1,190,476	0
Year 20	0	753,778
Net benefit, undiscounted ($)	250,000	1,000,000
Net benefit, discounted at 5% ($)	190,476	−246,222

Without discounting, the policymakers would conclude that both programs were desirable—each yields benefits in excess of what it costs—and Program 2 would be viewed as better than Program 1, since Program 2 produces net benefits (undiscounted benefits minus costs) of $1,000,000, while Program 1 produces net benefits of $250,000. But note what happens when we discount the benefits at 5 percent per year. The present value of Program 1's benefits equals $1,190,476 [$1,250,000/(1.05)]. The present value of Program 2's benefits equals $753, 778 [$2,000,000/(1.05)^{20}]. Thus, discounting at 5 percent, Program 1 now appears preferable to Program 2 because its discounted benefit is larger. Furthermore, Program 2 is no longer desirable because the present discounted value of its net benefit is negative: [$753,778 − $1,000,000 = −$246,222]. In other words, the *present value* of the future benefits is less than the cost of Program 2.

It is important to emphasize that discounting is *not* a device to correct for inflation. The preceding discussion assumed constant dollars, that is, it assumed that figures were presented in terms of the value of the dollar in a single year. Future dollar figures that are higher owing solely to inflation should be deflated by the rate of inflation *before* the discounting process begins. Discounting is intended to reflect the real opportunity cost of resources, not simply changes in the value of the currency.

COST ANALYSIS OF LIFETIME DENTAL CARE

This exercise will take a narrow view of dental-care costs. The "costs" of dental treatment, in fact, have been limited to direct expenditures. We have not included costs such as the value of time to the patient receiving care. We have made no attempt to put a monetary value on intangibles such as the cost of dental pain or the benefit of intact, healthy teeth. These are real costs and real benefits, but will have to be considered as value judgments in the final analysis.

Our approach has four sequential steps:

1. *To identify either those preventive procedures known to produce long-term benefits or those that appear most likely to do so.* Obviously a procedure must be effective if it is to have any cost-containment potential. Preventive techniques considered were those for caries and periodontal disease, in view of the absence of clearly defined primary prevention for other dental conditions such as malocclusion and clefts. As described earlier, it was not possible to check all preventive procedures. Those chosen for testing were water

fluoridation and regular professional cleanings as defined by Lindhe and Axelsson.[43] It is understood that control of periodontal disease cannot be expected without maintenance of a good level of oral hygiene by the individual.[44] Indeed, a high level of self-care is an integral part of the Swedish approach. It is assumed in these cost streams that the absence of a high level of oral hygiene will lead sooner or later to loss of teeth from periodontal disease.

2. *Development of seven streams of lifetime dental-care costs under different conditions.* A "cost stream" in this project is defined as the sequence of annual expenditures for dental care over the lifetime of a hypothetical individual. By using different combinations of various preventive procedures, and assuming different costs of some of them, the following seven cost streams were defined for hypothetical patients A through G who commence care at age six and complete it at age seventy-nine. Treatment is considered in five-year blocks to make the quantification more manageable.

A. A patient who totally neglects his/her oral health and receives only relief-of-pain extractions. The patient becomes edentulous soon after age thirty-five. Full dentures are provided then, and twice again during the age periods fifty to fifty-four and sixty-five to sixty-nine.

B. A patient who grows up with fluoridated water, receives regular care throughout life, but whose dentist is not oriented toward the control of periodontal disease. The patient receives no special periodontal care beyond periodic prophylaxes and eventually becomes edentulous between ages seventy to seventy-four.

C. The same patient as B, except that the patient does not grow up using fluoridated water. Attending the same dentist, and not having received the benefits of fluoridation, this patient becomes edentulous between the ages of fifty-five to fifty-nine.

D. A patient who grows up with fluoridated water and receives regular attention throughout life by a dentist who provides intensive periodontal care in the form of quarterly professional cleanings as defined by Lindhe and Axelsson.[45] As a result, the patient, who has lost only one tooth before age thirty-five, loses no more teeth thereafter. The dentist's excellent care, however, is provided at high fee levels.

E. The same patient as D, except that the patient does not grow up using fluoridated water. Patient E attends the same dentist. These factors mean that Patient E loses only three teeth before age thirty-five and none thereafter.

F. The same patient as D, except that the intensive periodontal care is provided by an auxiliary at lower fee levels. It is assumed in this project that the outcome of the treatment is the same as when the dentist provides the care.

G. The same patient as E, except that again the intensive periodontal care is provided by an auxiliary at lower fee levels than those of the dentist. Again, the outcome is assumed to be the same.

For this project, we took the patients in cost streams D through G who had been receiving annual maintenance care from ages six to twenty-four, and added the following regimens of periodontal treatment for their adult years, twenty-five to seventy-nine. A good level of personal hygiene is assumed throughout.

1. From ages twenty-five to thirty-four, four sessions per year (twenty per five-year period) of oral-hygiene instruction and reinforcement, plus one professional cleaning[46] annually during that period. The fee for the instruction sessions was assumed to be the same as for a prophylaxis ($15.35 in 1977[47]). The fee for the professional cleaning was taken as that for a periodontal scaling and root planing ($63.11 in 1977[48]) for the patients in cost streams D and E, and as that for a prophylaxis ($15.35) for patients in cost streams F and G.

2. From ages 34-79, four professional cleanings per year, that is at three-month intervals, twenty cleanings per five-year period. Again, the fee for these cleanings was $63.11 for those in cost streams D and E, and $15.35 for those in cost streams F and G.

These seven hypothetical lists of lifetime dental treatment received are summarized in table 3. Full details of treatment assumptions and the basis for them are given in the Appendix.

3. *Determination of the undiscounted costs of treatment.* The fee assessed for each item of treatment received was taken from mean fees given by general practitioners in the ADA's 1977 Survey of Dental Practice.[49] In each cost stream, lifetime dental expenditures were assessed by summing the fees for each item of service received. These undiscounted dollar values of care received over a lifetime are shown in table 4.

4. *Discounting the lifetime costs of treatment.* Finally, the expenditures shown in table 4 were discounted at an arbitrarily chosen rate of 4 percent; the results are also shown in table 4.

Results of the Project:

We have to make the point again that in this exercise we are dealing only with direct expenditures on dental care, rather than with total

Table 3. Major Dental Treatment Aspects of Seven Cost Streams

Aspects of dental treatment	Cost streams						
	A	B	C	D	E	F	G
Fluoridated water supply	No	Yes	No	Yes	No	Yes	No
Annual topical fluorides to age 24	No	No	Yes	No	Yes	No	Yes
Visits for dental treatment	At ages 7, 12, 18, 21, 35, 45, 65	Annually to age 29; 3 per 5 years. ages 30-59; 2 per 5 yrs. ages 60-79	Annually to age 29; 3 per 5 yrs. ages 30-59; once ages 60-64	Annually to age 79			
Prophylaxes	No	Same schedule as visits for treatment		Annually to age 24			
Professional cleaning*	No	No			Annually ages 25-34; Quarterly ages 35-79		
Cost of professional cleaning	—		—	High, same as periodontal scaling		Low, same as prophylaxis	
Tooth loss history	5 by age 24; 15 by age 34; all by 35-39	3 by age 44; 12 by age 59; all by 70-74	1 by age 24; 10 by age 44; all by 55-59	1 by age 34; no more	3 by age 34; no more	1 by age 34; no more	3 by age 34; no more
Bridges	No	1 by age 44	1 by age 29; 2 by age 44	1 by age 39	1 by age 29; 2 by age 39	1 by age 39	1 by age 29; 2 by age 39
Partial dentures	No	1 PU by 50-54; 1 PL by 60-64	1 PU by 45-49; 1 PL by 50-54	No			
Full upper and full lower dentures	By ages 35-39	By ages 70-74	By ages 55-59	No			

*Professional cleaning is as defined by Per Axelsson and Jan Lindhe, "The Effect of a Preventive Programme on Dental Plaque, Gingivitis and Caries in Schoolchildren: Results After One and Two Years," *Journal of Clinical Periodontology* 1(2), pp. 126-38, 1974.

costs. What we have arrived at is a series of total direct expenditures under different conditions and with different outcomes. The eventual decision on what is the "best buy" is essentially a value judgment.

The final caveat here is that there is no adjustment for inflation. The only difference this introduces is that the total discounted costs shown in table 4 may seem extremely small to many. Perhaps the best way of visualizing these amounts is to think of them as the expenditures required now, in 1977 dollars, for a one-time payment for dental treatment to be provided throughout life.

The results in table 4 show that the cheapest form of dental treatment is that for cost stream A, in which there was total neglect. According to the model, total neglect (or no prevention at all) costs $2,745 less than the most expensive cost stream, E, or about one-third as much in direct expenditures. But total neglect is only $847, in discounted 1977 dollars, less expensive than cost stream C, about 60 percent of the price. Cost stream C, it will be recalled, is the patient on nonfluoridated water who receives regular treatment in youth,

Table 4. Dollar Value of Dental Care Received in Undiscounted and Discounted 1977 Dollars per Five-Year Period from Ages 6 to 79, for Patients in Each of the Seven Cost Streams

Age Groups	Undiscounted Value of Care Received in Each Cost Stream A-G ($)						
	A	B	C	D	E	F	G
6-9	182	295	402	295	402	295	402
10-14	288	342	409	342	409	342	409
15-19	389	403	458	403	458	403	458
20-24	426	465	528	465	528	465	528
25-29	0	159	802	701	1,329	199	792
30-34	153	126	161	717	736	214	233
35-39	819	126	176	1,925	1,944	947	966
40-44	0	719	769	1,332	1,352	389	408
45-49	0	157	456	1,332	1,352	389	408
50-54	559	437	399	1,332	1,352	389	408
55-59	0	157	677	1,332	1,352	389	408
60-64	0	375	153	1,332	1,352	389	408
65-69	559	94	0	1,332	1,352	389	408
70-74	0	729	0	1,332	1,352	389	408
75-79	0	153	0	1,332	1,352	389	408
Totals in undiscounted 1977 dollars	3,375	4,737	5,390	15,504	16,622	5,977	7,052
Totals in dollars discounted at 4%	1,273	1,568	2,120	3,504	4,018	1,856	2,355

but no special periodontal care and loses all teeth by age fifty-five to fifty-nine.

The results also suggest that water fluoridation does reduce expenditures. Cost stream B is cheaper than C by $552 (or 74 percent as much); D is $514 less than E (or 87 percent as much), and F is $499 less than G (or 79 percent as much). Regardless, therefore, of additional treatment expenditures, this model suggests that water fluoridation results in substantial reductions in direct expenditures for dental treatment over a lifetime.

The addition of intensive periodontal treatment provided by the dentist at high fees obviously results in greater expenditures. Cost streams D and E, fluoridated and nonfluoridated areas with the expensive periodontal treatment in addition, are $1,384 (165 percent) and $1,898 (190 percent) more expensive than cost stream C. Where the intensive periodontal treatment with the same outcome can be provided less expensively by an auxiliary, as in cost streams F and G, results are much closer to those in cost stream C. The patient in cost stream F, with fluoridated water, spends $264 less than the patient in cost stream C, or only 88 percent as much. The patient in cost stream G, without fluoridation, spends $235 more than (or 111 percent of) the patient in cost stream C.

Discussion: Sensitivity Analysis

Any modeling exercise of this nature is based on explicit and implicit assumptions. Acceptance of conclusions reached is, therefore, conditioned by the degree of acceptance of these assumptions. Economics modeling often includes "sensitivity analysis," which is a method of testing the importance of the assumptions by changing each one in turn and holding all other factors in the model constant. If the use of a different assumed value does not change the qualitative conclusions reached, then the assumption is not all that important; the model is not "sensitive" to the use of different values for that particular assumption. If, however, changes in assumed values do lead to changes in conclusions, that is if the model is "sensitive" to the use of different values for a particular assumption, then it is clear that whatever value is selected for the assumption is important. Sensitivity analysis does not tell the researcher what values should or should not be selected for use in the model, only which are the more critical assumptions. Discount values selected, for example, are often critical in economic models, although they were not in this one. While 4 percent was the value chosen that leads to the results in table 4, the model was also tested with discount values of 2 percent and 6 percent. The rankings of the cost streams did not change.

Full sensitivity analysis was not carried out in this model. Areas worth examining would include the benefit of fluoridation; effectiveness of routine prophylaxis and of the intensive priodontal care throughout life; the likely treatment plans in each cost stream; and the possibility of different dental-health outcomes with the auxiliary treatment in cost streams F and G.

Discussion: Implications of Results

It is worth considering Holtzman's cautions on hopes for prevention as a cost-containment strategy in health care.[50] It is Holtzman's belief that the cost-containment prospect for prevention is less than that frequently promised and that campaigns for changes in lifestyle are likely to have most effect in those with the lightest burden of illness. Applying these cautionary thoughts to dentistry, we might conclude that total prevention of disease over a lifetime is probably impossible for most people. But what is possible for many of these same people is substantial prevention of caries and control of periodontal disease to a point where inflammation is minor and loss of bony support is minimized. If this relatively limited goal can be accepted, then the nature of lifetime prevention in a cost-containment context perhaps becomes clearer.

One approach to the task of assessing the cost-containment potential of prevention would have been to define a standard outcome in several different cost streams, such as a particular number of teeth lost at a particular age, and then to judge the various alternative ways of reaching it. We chose the approach we did, with four different outcomes in seven cost streams, to allow the exercise of some value judgments in determining which options might be preferable, for there are clear tradeoffs to be made between cost and quality of outcome.

The cheapest form of prevention is total neglect, doing nothing until forced to, using no preventive or even restorative services at all and losing all teeth at an early age. Some individuals no doubt still live this way, but it cannot be offered as an acceptable option for the vast majority of the population. Values intrude and in the United States it is a widely held value that retention of teeth, at least through middle age, is socially and culturally desirable. However, the results of this simulation suggest that total neglect requires the lowest expenditures of all the cost streams examined. The addition of any prevention at all will require more. On the other hand, to reiterate the point made at the beginning of this chapter, we have not taken into account the costs of pain, poor appearance, and loss of quality of life. In the case of the patient in cost stream A, these are likely to be considerable.

Two of the cost streams (B and C) have assumed eventual loss of all teeth, mostly because of periodontal disease and the absence of special steps to prevent it. This outcome of total tooth loss was included because it still does occur and because there clearly are implications for lifetime expenditures on dental treatment. Cost stream B, in which the benefits of fluoridation delayed total tooth loss until late in life, was the second least expensive cost stream, but total tooth loss did eventually occur. (The cost of the fluoridation process was not included in the analysis because it is so low[51] that it can be left out.)

Probably cost stream F would seem to most in dentistry as the most desirable option. It is $288 more expensive (18 percent) than cost stream B in discounted 1977 dollars, but it assumes almost total tooth retention as against total tooth loss. Is it worth $288 to save teeth? Dentists no doubt think so; what about the public? Perhaps it should be pointed out again that the relatively low expenditures in cost stream F were achieved because a lesser-trained auxiliary was used, and the assumption was made that the quality of the auxiliary's care was similar to that of the dentist's.

There are some unaccounted-for costs for the patient in cost stream F that should be emphasized. We have allowed regular annual visits to age thirty-four, then a regular pattern of four visits annually from thirty-five to seventy-nine. Not many individuals, we suggest, would adhere scrupulously to such a pattern, and if they did there would obviously be costs to the patient. The more that an individual deviates from that pattern, the less favorable the outcome is likely to be. If some teeth are lost, either more dental treatment will be required or the quality of life will be diminished.

Several implications emerge from this exercise. One, fairly free of value judgments, is that water fluoridation is likely to reduce the costs (all costs) of dental care, of and by itself. As a community measure, the costs of water fluoridation are largely in its installation; operating costs are low. So long as the estimates of dental-health benefits used in this exercise can be accepted, fluoridation can be accepted as having cost-containment potential.

The regimen of professional cleanings and personal oral hygiene does not provide such unequivocal benefits. Assuming that it is as effective as we have allowed for, its cost-containment potential is related to the dental status desired. Repeating a statement made in our introduction that seems appropriate here, the cost-containment potential of a prevention activity is rarely independent of the intensity with which it is pursued.

CONCLUSIONS

Within the limitations of the study method, the following conclusions can be presented:

- Total neglect is the least expensive form of dental care in terms of direct dental-care expenditures.
- Water fluoridation reduces the cost of dental care over a lifetime.
- Assuming that regular professional cleanings and patient education four times per year in adulthood minimize tooth loss, the expense of achieving this outcome is reduced if the cleanings can be provided at low fee levels and if the benefits of fluoridation are also available.
- Maximum oral-health benefits of regular professional periodontal care may have implications for development of new dental auxiliaries and of different delivery systems. If so, the full cost-containment potential of prevention cannot be assessed independently of the implications for education and delivery systems.
- Because different combinations of preventive care are likely to result in different oral-health outcomes, value judgments are still required to determine the best options in applying the cost-containing potential of preventive procedures.

Appendix

Details of Lifetime Dental Treatment

This project required definition of dental treatment received over a lifetime, under different conditions, so that the cost-containment potential of various preventive procedures could be assessed. Data available in the dental literature are limited to treatment provided to specific groups, usually over a short period of time. While such data are useful in making projections, there are still numerous assumptions which have to be made.

The seven cost streams were fully defined in the chapter section, Cost Analysis of Lifetime Dental Care, above. The first stream was the total neglect patient. The second and third were identical except that one received the benefits of fluoridated water and the other did not. The fourth and fifth streams were the same as the second and third, except the patients

Table A1. Number of Dental Service Items Received by Children and Young Adults Who Have Received Fluoridated Water All Their Lives

Service item	6-9	10-14	15-19	20-24
Examination	4	5	5	5
Prophylaxis	4	5	5	5
Topical fluoride	4	5	5	5
Radiographs FS	2	2	2	2
Radiographs BW	2	3	3	3
Perm. 1-surf. am.	0.74	1.50	0.88	0.95
Perm. 2-surf. am.	—*	0.17	0.87	0.72
Perm. 3-surf. am.	—	—	0.41	0.6
Porcelain/metal crown	—	—	0.06	0.8
Post crown	—	—	0.1	0.13
3-unit bridge	—	—	0	0
Prim. 1-surf. am.	1.48	0.01	—	—
Prim. 2-surf. am.	0.93	0.01	—	—
Prim. 3-surf. am.	0.19	—	—	—
Stainless steel crown	0.18	—	—	—
Extractions	0.28	0.03	0.04	0.05
Perio Scale/root plane	—	0.09	0.16	0.26
Gingivectomy/flap	—	0.05	0.1	0.13
Space maintainers	0.03	—	—	—
Interceptive ortho	0.08	0.13	—	—
Pulpotomy	0.05	—	—	—
Anterior RCT	—	0.15	0.2	0.25
Molar RCT	—	—	—	—
Partial denture	—	—	0.01	0.03
FU/FL dentures	—	—	—	—
FU dentures	—	—	—	—
Impacted tooth extr.	—	—	0.12	0.2

Source: B. A Burt, A Method of Comparing the Expenditures on Two Alternative National Dental Programs for Persons Aged 6-21, Final Report, USPHS Contract No. N01-DH-44101 (Ann Arbor, Mich.: University of Michigan, 1975), pp. 64-75.

*Dashes stand for absolute zero; zeroes mean less than 0.01.

received extensive periodontal care from a dentist throughout life. Patients in the sixth and seventh streams received identical treatment to the fourth and fifth, except that their equally effective periodontal treatments were provided by auxiliaries at lower fee levels.

Treatment received by children and young adults had been described in detail in previous publications,[52] and is repeated here in tables A1 and A2. The same information was used in this project. These tables were based on available data to the extent possible to determine disease increments and treatment received. Guidelines from the American Dental Association,[53] and the American Academy of Pedodontics, and the American Society of Dentistry for Children[54] were employed to determine service requirements.

Principal restrictions employed in determining service requirements up to age twenty-four were:

Table A2. Number of Dental Service Items Received by Children and Young Adults Who Have Received Nonfluoridated Water All Their Lives

Service item	6-9	10-14	15-19	20-24
Examination	4	5	5	5
Prophylaxis	4	5	5	5
Topical fluoride	4	5	5	5
Radiographs FS	2	2	2	2
Radiographs BW	2	3	3	3
Perm. 1-surf. am.	1.36	1.15	1.18	1.4
Perm. 2-surf. am.	—*	1.28	1.14	1.3
Perm. 3-surf. am.	—	—	0.53	0.85
Porcelain/metal crown	—	—	0.06	0.08
Post crown	—	—	0.1	0.13
3-unit bridge	—	—	0	0
Prim. 1-surf. am.	3.29	0.08	—	—
Prim. 2-surf. am.	2.02	0.04	—	—
Prim. 3-surf. am.	0.45	0.01	—	—
Stainless steel crown	0.23	—	—	—
Extractions	0.57	0.28	0.32	0.4
Perio Scale/root plane	—	0.09	0.19	0.26
Gingivectomy/flap	—	0.05	0.1	0.13
Space maintainers	0.14	—	—	—
Interceptive ortho	0.1	0.13	—	—
Pulpotomy	—	—	—	—
Anterior RCT	—	0.2	0.25	0.25
Molar RCT	—	—	—	—
Partial denture	—	—	0.01	0.03
FU/FL dentures	—	—	—	—
FU dentures	—	—	—	—
Impacted tooth extr.	—	—	0.12	0.2

Source: B. A Burt, *A Method of Comparing the Expenditures on Two Alternative National Dental Programs for Persons Aged 6-21*, Final Report, USPHS Contract No. N01-DH-44101 (Ann Arbor, Mich.: University of Michigan, 1975), pp. 64-75.

*Dashes stand for absolute zero; zeroes mean less than 0.01.

1. Orthodontic care would be restricted to space maintainers and simple interceptive care of up to six months' duration.
2. No gold restorations, or any kind of restoration in primary anterior teeth, would be used.
3. Treatment of primary teeth would cease at age twelve.
4. Full-series radiographs would be taken every three years, bitewings in the intervening years.
5. No consideration was given to acid-etch procedures, major oral surgery, or repair of cleft lip and palate.

It was also assumed that children in fluoridated areas received full benefit from fluoridation, those in nonfluoridated areas no benefit, although they would receive some benefits from the annual topical fluoride. Treatment received from ages twenty-two to twenty-four was assumed to be the same as that received at age twenty-one.

Treatment received by the hypothetical patients, showing total numbers of services received from six to nine and then in five-year blocks from age ten to twenty-four, are shown in tables A1 and A2. The patients are those receiving annual maintenance care in a fluoridated area (table A1, cost streams B, D, and F) and annual maintenance care in a nonfluoridated area (table A2, cost streams C, E, and G).

Treatment received by the patient who is neglecting his or her oral health is confined to extractions, which number five by age twenty-four, a further 10 at ages thirty to thirty-four, and the final seventeen at ages thirty-five to thirty-nine, at which time full upper and lower dentures are inserted. A new set of dentures is made at age fifty to fifty-four, and a third set provided at ages sixty-five to sixty-nine. Treatment for the patient in cost stream A is not tabulated in table A3, but is summarized in table 2 in the main text.

Table A3. Number of Dental-Service Items Received for Adults in Cost Streams B-E.

Age Groups	B	C	D	E
25-29	5 examinations 5 prophylaxes 2 replacements (2 surf. amalgams)	5 examinations 5 prophylaxes 3 replacements (2 surf. amalgams) 2 extractions 1 3-unit bridge	5 examinations 5 prof. cleanings 20 O.H. instructions 2 replacements (2 surf. amalgams)	5 examinations 5 prof. cleanings 20 O.H. instructions 3 replacements (2 surf. amalgams) 1 extraction 1 3-unit bridge
30-34	3 examinations 3 prophylaxes 2 replacements (2 surf. amalgams) 1 extraction	3 examinations 3 prophylaxes 3 replacements (2 surf. amalgams) 2 extractions	5 examinations 5 prof. cleanings 20 O.H. instructions 2 replacements (2 surf. amalgams) 1 extraction	5 examinations 5 prof. cleanings 20 O.H. instructions 3 replacements (2 surf. amalgams) 1 extraction
35-39	3 examinations 3 prophylaxes 2 replacements (2 surf. amalgams) 1 extraction	3 examinations 3 prophylaxes 3 replacements (2 surf. amalgams) 3 extractions	5 examinations 20 prof. cleanings 2 replacements (2 surf. amalgams) 1 3-unit bridge	5 examinations 20 prof. cleanings 3 replacements (2 surf. amalgams) 1 3-unit bridge
40-44	3 examinations 3 prophylaxes 2 replacements (2 surf. amalgams) 1 extraction 1 3-unit bridge	3 examinations 3 prophylaxes 3 replacements (2 surf. amalgams) 3 extractions 1 3-unit bridge	5 examinations 20 prof. cleanings 2 replacements (2 surf. amalgams)	5 examinations 20 prof. cleanings 3 replacements (2 surf. amalgams)
45-49	3 examinations 3 prophylaxes 2 replacements (2 surf. amalgams) 3 extractions	3 examinations 3 prophylaxes 3 replacements (2 surf. amalgams) 3 extractions 1 part upper denture	Same as ages 40-44	Same as ages 40-44

Table A3 — *Continued*

Age Groups	B	C	D	E
50-54	3 examinations 3 prophylaxes 2 replacements (2 surf. amalgams) 3 extractions 1 part upper denture	3 examinations 3 prophylaxes 3 extractions 1 part lower denture	Same as ages 40-44	Same as ages 40-44
55-59	3 examinations 3 prophylaxes 2 replacements (2 surf. amalgams)	3 examinations 6 extractions Full upper and lower dentures	Same as ages 40-44	Same as ages 40-44
60-64	2 examinations 2 prophylaxes 3 extractions 1 part lower denture	1 reline (FU/FL dentures)	Same as ages 40-44	Same as ages 40-44
65-69	2 examinations 2 prophylaxes 3 extractions	NONE	Same as ages 40-44	Same as ages 40-44
70-74	2 examinations 10 extractions Full upper and full lower dentures	NONE	Same as ages 40-44	Same as ages 40-44
75-79	1 reline (FU/FL dentures)	NONE	Same as ages 40-44	Same as ages 40-44

Note: Patients in cost streams F and G receive the same service items as those in D and E, but the fees for periodontal care are different.

The extreme detail in tables A1 and A2 was used because these tables were taken from an existing source. No such source existed for adults older than twenty-five, so treatment plans had to be developed for continuation of the patients in tables A1 and A2. Because of the complexity of treatment required in adults, the plans were kept relatively simple. These philosophies guided the development of treatment plans:

1. The hypothetical patients in cost streams B and C continue to receive regular care, though it becomes less than annual visits after age twenty-nine. (Schedule of visits in table 2.) Neither patient receives any special periodontal treatment or instructions beyond prophylaxes at each visit. As a result, periodontal disease become established and progressive tooth loss sets in, an outcome periodontists consider likely.[55] The patient in cost stream C, without fluoridation, becomes edentulous at ages fifty-five to fifty-nine. The patient in cost stream B, with fluoridation, becomes edentulous at ages seventy to seventy-four. It is assumed that periodontal disease progresses at the same rate in both patients. The benefits of fluoridation, however, have allowed the patient in cost stream B to retain teeth approximately fifteen years longer.

2. The patients in cost streams D and E are the same as those in B and C, except that they receive intensive preventive periodontal care throughout life. It is assumed that this treatment is successful in preventing any further tooth loss after age thirty-five.

158   Burt and Warner

The periodontal care by intensive professional cleaning[56] is provided expensively, here defined as the fee equivalent to a periodontal scaling and root planing in 1977 ($63.11).[57]

3. Patients in cost streams F and G have exactly the same history as those in D and E, except that the professional cleanings are provided less expensively, in this case for a fee equivalent to a prophylaxis in 1977 ($15.35[58]).

For the sake of simplicity, no radiographs, gold restorations, crowns, endodontics, or orthodontics are included in care received from age twenty-five to seventy-nine. The fee for oral hygiene instruction and reinforcement (ages twenty-five to thirty-four, cost streams D-G) is taken as the same as for a prophylaxis ($15.35). It is assumed that such care is part of the intensive periodontal treatment (ages thirty-five to seventy-nine, cost streams D-G) and is provided only cursorily, if at all, for patients in cost streams B and C.

Notes

1. B. A. Burt. "Tentative Analysis of the Efficiency of a Fissure Sealant in a Public Program in London," *Community Dentistry Oral Epidemiology*, 5, (2), 1977:73-77.

2. American Dental Association, Bureau of Economic Research and Statistics. *Prescribing and Dispensing Habits of Dentists, 1975*. (Chicago: ADA, 1976), pp. 6-7.

3. H. C. Gift, and B. B. Milton. "Comparison of Two National Preventive Dentistry Surveys: 1957 and 1974." Abstr. 158, Annual session of the American Association for Dental Research, *J. Dent. Res.*, 54, (Spec. Issue A), 1975:84.

4. F. J. Margolis, et al. "A Survey of Physicians' Prescriptions of Fluoride Supplements for Their Child Patients," *Am. J. Dis. Child.*, 134, (9), 1980, 865-868.

5. American Dental Association, Bureau of Economic Research and Statistics. *The 1977 Survey of Dental Practice*. (Chicago: ADA, 1978), pp. 23-26.

6. R. C. Faine. "An Agenda for the Eighties: Community and School Fluoridation," *J. Pub. Health Dent.*, 40, (3), 1980, 258-267.

7. A. M. Horowitz. "An Agenda for the Eighties: Self-Applied Fluorides," *J. Pub. Health Dent.*, 40, (3), 1980, 268-275.

8. Gift and Milton, "Comparison of Surveys," p. 84.

9. D. Jackson. "Dental Caries: the Distinction between Delay and Prevention," *Brit. Dent. J.*, 137, (9), 1974:347-351.

10. F. Brudevold and R. Naujoks. "Caries-Preventive Fluoride Treatment for the Individual," *Caries Res.* 12 (Suppl. 1), 1978:52-64.

11. B. A. Burt, ed. *The Relative Efficiency of Methods of Caries Prevention in Dental Public Health*. Proceedings of a workshop at the University of Michigan, June 5-8, 1978. (Ann Arbor: University of Michigan, 1979.)

12. O. Backer Dirks, W. Kunzel, and J. P. Carlos. "Caries-Preventive Water Fluoridation," *Caries Res.*, 12 (Suppl. 1), 1978:7-14.

13. Burt, *The Relative Efficiency*.

14. G. N. Davies. *Cost and Benefit of Fluoride in the Prevention of Dental Caries*. (Geneva: World Health Organization Offset Publication No. 9, 1974.); W. Nelson and J. M. Swint. "Cost-Benefit Analysis of Fluoridation in Houston, Texas," *J. Pub. Health Dent.*, 36, (2), 1976:88-95; T. B. Dowell. "The Economics of Fluoridation," *Brit. Dent. J.*, 140, (3), 1977:103-106; D. P. Doessel. *A Cost Benefit Analysis of Water Fluoridation in Townsville: A Report to the Economic and Financial Research Fund of the Reserve Bank of Australia*. (Brisbane, Aust.: Univ. Queensland, 1977.); P. E. Fidler. "A Comparison of Treatment Patterns and Costs for a Fluoride and Non-Fluoride Community," *Community Health,*

9, (2), 1978:103-113; E. Newburn. "Cost Effectiveness and Practicality Features in the Systemic Use of Fluorides," in B. A. Burt, ed. *The Relative Efficiency.*

15. D. B. Ast, N. C. Cons, S. T. Pollard, and J. Garfinkel. "Time and Cost Factors to Provide Regular, Periodic Dental Care for Children in a Fluoridated and Non-Fluoridated Area: Final Report," *Am. Dent. A. J.*, 80, (4), 1970:770-776; N. Doherty and E. Powell. "Effects of Age and Years of Exposure on the Economic Benefits of Fluoridation," *J. Dent. Res.*, 53, (8), 1974:912-914.

16. D. Jackson, J. J. Murray, and C. G. Fairpo. "Life-Long Benefits of Fluoride in Drinking Water," *Brit. Dent. J.*, 134, (10), 1973:419-422.

17. H. R. Englander and D. A. Wallace. "Effects of Naturally Fluoridated Water on Dental Caries in Adults," *Pub. Health Rep.* 77, (10), 1962:887-893.

18. A. L. Russell and Elias Elvove. "Domestic Water and Dental Caries. VII. A Study of the Fluoride-Dental Caries Relationship in an Adult Population," *Pub. Health Rep.*, 66, (9), 1951:1389-1401.

19. J. J. Murray. "Adult Dental Health in Fluoride and Non-Fluoride Areas. Part 1 — Mean DMF Values by Age," *Brit. Dent. J.*, 131. (9), 1971:391-395; J. J. Murray. "Adult Dental Health in Fluoride and Non-Fluoride Areas. Part 3 — Tooth Mortality by Age," *Brit. Dent. J.*, 131, (11), 1971:487-492.

20. A. L. Russell. "Fluoride Domestic Water and Periodontal Disease," *Am. J. Pub. Health*, 47, (6), 1957:688-694.

21. J. W. Stamm and D. W. Banting. "Comparison of Root Caries Prevalence in Adults with Life-Long Residence in Fluoridated and Non-Fluoridated Communities." Abstr. No. 552, Annual session of the American Association for Dental Research, *J. Dent. Res.*, 59 (Spec. Issue A, 405).

22. S. B. Heifetz, H. S. Horowitz, and W. S. Driscoll. "Effect of School Water Fluoridation on Dental Caries: Results in Seagrove, N.C., after 8 Years," *Am. Dent. A. J.*, 97, (2), 1978:193-196.

23. T. M. Marthaler, et al. "Caries Preventive Salt Fluoridation," *Caries Res.* 12 (Suppl. 1), 1978:15-21.

24. W. S. Driscoll. "The Use of Fluoride Tablets for the Prevention of Dental Caries," in D. J. Forrester, and E. M. Schulz, Jr. *International Workshop on Fluorides.* (Baltimore: University of Maryland, 1974.); W. S. Driscoll, S. B. Heifetz, and D. C. Korts. "Effect of Chewable Fluoride Tablets on Dental Caries in Schoolchildren: Results after Six Years of Use," *Am. Dent. A. J.*, 97, (5), 1978:820-824.

25. F. Brudevold and R. Naujoks, "Caries-Preventive Fluoride Treatment."

26. S. B. Heifetz. "Cost-Effectiveness of Topically-Applied Fluorides," in B. A. Burt, ed., *The Relative Efficiency.*

27. A. M. Horowitz, "An Agenda for the Eighties," p. 268-275.

28. H. S. Horowitz, et al. "Evaluation of a Combination or Self-Administered Fluoride Procedure for the Control of Dental Caries in a Non-Fluoride Area: Findings after Four Years," *Am. Dent. A. J.*, 98, (2), 1979:219-223.

29. H. R. Englander, et al. "Incremental Rates of Dental Caries after Repeated Sodium Fluoride Applications in Children with Lifelong Consumption of Fluoridated Water," *Am. Dent. A. J.*, 82, (2), 1971:354-358; S. B. Heifetz, et al. "Combined Anticariogenic Effect of Fluoride Gel-Grays and Fluoride Mouthrinsing in an Optimally Fluoridated Community," *J. Clin. Prev. Dent.*, 6, (1), 1979:21-23, 28.

30. F. R. Von der Fehr and I. J. Moller. "Caries-Preventive Fluoride Dentifrices," *Caries Res.* 12, (Suppl. 1):31-37.

31. Brudevold and Naujoks, "Caries-Preventive Fluoride Treatment"; Horowitz and M. C. Kau. "Retained Anticaries Protection from Topically Applied Acidulated Phosphate-Fluoride 30- and 36-Month Post-Treatment Effects," *J. Prevent. Dent.*, 1, (1), 1974:22-27.

32. Brudevold and Naujoks, "Caries-Preventive Fluoride Treatment"; W. S. Driscoll, S. B. Heifetz, and J. A. Brunelle. "Treatment and Post-Treatment Effects of Chewable Fluoride Tablets on Dental Caries: Results after 7½ Years," *Am. Dent. A. J.*, 99, (5), 1979:817-821.

33. Burt, *The Relative Efficiency*.

34. *Ibid*.

35. H. Loe, A. Anerud, H. Boysen, and M. Smith, "The Natural History of Periodontal Disease in Man. Study Design and Baseline Data," *J. Periodont. Res.*, 13, (6), 1978:550-562; Loe, et al., "The Natural History of Periodontal Disease in Man. The Rate of Periodontal Destruction before 40 Years of Age," *J. Periodont. Res.*, 49, (12), 1978:607-620; A. Anerud, H. Loe, H. Boysen, and M. Smith. "The Natural History of Periodontal Disease in Man. Changes in Gingival Health and Oral Hygiene before 40 Years of Age," *J. Periodont. Res.*, 14, (6), 1979:526-540.

36. A. Sheiham. "Prevention and Control of Periodontal Disease," in *International Conference on Research in the Biology of Periodontal Disease*. Univ. of Illinois College of Dentistry, Chicago, June 12-15, 1977.

37. P. Axelsson and J. Lindhe, "The Effect of a Preventive Programme on Dental Plaque, Gingivitis and Caries in Schoolchildren. Results after One and Two Years," *J. Clin. Periodontol*, 1, (2), 1974:126-138; P. Axelsson, J. Lindhe, and J. Waseby. "The Effect of Various Plaque Control Measures on Gingivitis and Caries in Schoolchildren," *Community Dent. Oral Epidemiol.*, 4, (6), 1976:232-239; P. Axelsson and J. Lindhe. "Effect of a Plaque Control Program on Gingivitis and Dental Caries in Schoolchildren," *J. Dent. Res.* 56 (Spec. Issue C), 1977:c142-c148.

38. P. Axelsson and J. Lindhe. "Effect of Controlled Oral Procedures on Caries and Periodontal Disease in Adults," *J. Clin. Periodontol.*, 5, (2), 1978:133-151.

39. B. Rosling, S. Nyman, and J. Lindhe. "The Effect of Systematic Plaque Control on Bone Regeneration in Infrabony Pockets," *J. Clin. Periodontol.*, 3, (1), 1976:38-53.

40. S. P. Ramfjord, J. W. Knowles, R. R. Nissle, R. A. Schick, and F. G. Burgett. "Longitudinal Study of Periodontal Therapy," *J. Periodont.*, 44, (2), 1973:66-77; E. C. Morrison. *The Effect of Professional Prophylaxis and Personal Oral Hygiene on the Severity of Periodontitis*. Doctoral dissertation, the University of Michigan, Ann Arbor, 1977.

41. J. Ainamo. "Control of Plaque by Chemical Agents," *J. Clin. Periodontol.*, 4, 1977: 23-35.

42. Axelsson and Lindhe. "The Effect of a Preventive Programme."

43. *Ibid*.

44. Sheiham. "Prevention and Control."

45. Axelsson and Lindhe. "The Effect of a Preventive Programme."

46. *Ibid*.

47. American Dental Association, Bureau of Economic Research and Statistics. "Dental Fees Charged by General Practitioners and Selected Specialists in the United States," *Am. Dent. A. J.*, 97, (4), 678-690.

48. *Ibid*.

49. *Ibid*.

50. N. A. Holtzman. "Prevention: Rhetoric and Reality," *Internat. J. Health Services*, 9, (1), 1979:25-39.

51. Newbrun, "Cost-Effectiveness and Practicality Features in the Systematic Use of Fluorides, in B. A. Burt, ed., *The Relative Efficiency*.

52. Burt, "Diagnostic and Preventive Services in a National Incremental Plan for Children," *J. Pub. Health Dent.*, 37, (1), 1977:31-46. B. A. Burt, *A Method of Comparing the Expenditures on Two Alternative National Dental Programs for Persons Aged 6-21*. Final report, USPHS Contract No. N01-DH-44101. (Ann Arbor, Mich., 1975.), pp. 42-75.

53. American Dental Association, "Guidelines for Dentistry's Position in a National Health Program," *Am. Dent. A. J.*, 83, (6), 1971:1226-1232.

54. B. E. Johnson and W. O. Young, eds. *Manual for Children's Dental Care Programs*. 2nd ed. (Chicago: American Academy of Pedodontics and American Society of Dentistry for Children, 1974.)

55. "Committee Report on the Prevention and Control of Periodontal Disease," in *International Conference on Research in the Biology of Periodontal Disease*. (Chicago: Univ. of Illinois, College of Dentistry, June 12-15, 1977.)

56. Axelsson and Lindhe. "The Effect of a Preventive Programme."

57. American Dental Association. "Dental Fees Charged," pp. 678-690.

58. *Ibid*.

6

Quality Assurance

Marvin Marcus and Samuel J. Tobin

The relationship between quality and cost is never obvious. This relationship becomes more obscure when we are considering the behavior of a diverse system such as dental care. This chapter will probe the concepts of quality and quality-assurance systems. We will specifically explore the following areas: (1) problems concerning quality assurance, (2) components and types of quality assurance, (3) institutional circumstances that affect quality assurance, (4) interaction of costs, quality assurance, and problems of quality, and (5) examination of potential effectiveness of quality-assurance systems.

CONCEPTS AND LANGUAGE OF QUALITY OF CARE

Quality care results in an improvement in the individual's state of health and well-being. A problem arises when we try to define quality of care and then try to integrate it into policy. R. I. Lee and L. W. Jones in 1933 defined good medical care as that practiced and taught by recognized leaders of the medical profession.[1] This definition delegates quality judgments to the profession and ignores the consumer and the financial intermediary. R. H. Brook et al. divide the definition of quality into technical care and art of care.[2] Technical care refers to the provider's ability to produce the diagnostic and therapeutic care required by the patient. Art of care concerns more subtle dimensions

We thank Dr. Kent Nash for his insightful comments and the assistance he provided us. The model presented here was part of a PHS funded project, HRA Contract No. 231-77-0076, Dr. Howard Kelly, Project Officer. Finally, many thanks to Vera Snyder and Leslie Hanson for their help in producing this chapter.

of provider and system behavior such as promoting positive health habits, providing an environment conducive to patient care, and establishing interpersonal relationships with patients. Even though Donabedian alleges that use of the term "art of care" can be misleading, the interpersonal dimension is basic to any definition of quality.[3] For example, a dentist may produce a technically excellent bridge but fail to involve the patient in the appropriate home care to maintain the appliance. Because art of care is difficult to evaluate, most of the current activity centers on the technical aspects of quality. From a cost-containment perspective, technical care and art of care should be considered together in developing programs and policy.

The ability of the provider and the system to produce a level of quality for specific services brings us to the concepts of efficacy and effectiveness.[4] Efficacy refers to the benefit of a procedure performed under ideal conditions. An efficacious procedure in the hands of certain providers, however, could be ineffective. For example, we may all agree that a bridge is the treatment of choice in a certain situation. However, it is possible that the patient might be better off not receiving that service from some practitioners. In considering quality of care, it is necessary to recognize the potential gap between efficacy and effectiveness of treatment.

This naturally leads to the concept of criteria and standards. We may use Lee's and Jones's definitions of quality of care to establish the basis for what we would consider high-quality dental care. The guidelines of the California Dental Association's task force on quality are one example of a set of criteria that delineate four levels of quality.[5] These criteria are the basis for making judgments about the technical quality of care. Once the criteria have been defined, another perhaps more difficult set of decisions has to be made regarding the standards that are acceptable. A standard is the expected level of performance for a given criterion.[6] For example, if we accept that good endodontic therapy consists of asymptomatic filling of the root canals within 1 mm of the apex with a dense material, then do we require that all endodontic services must meet this criterion or can we accept some lower tolerance of performance? Setting the level of a standard is a function of complexity of the tasks involved in the procedure, risk to the patient if the criterion is not met, and the general level of performance in the community. The question of the level of the standard is crucial to deciding the quality issue.

We now turn from basic definitional concepts to discuss a framework for evaluation. Donabedian delineates the evaluation of care systems into structure, process, and outcome dimensions.[7] By structure, he refers to the organizational and material resources available to support the provision of care. A well-trained staff, good equipment, and management can be assumed to contribute to high-quality care.

But observing excellent structural elements is an insufficient basis for ensuring that the care is of high quality. The process dimension refers to the interactions between the patient and the system in terms of events that do or do not occur in the provision of care. Reviewing patient records for appropriateness of care and examining restorations for integrity of margins are examples of process-of-care evaluation approaches. Most quality-assurance activity is presently in the areas of structure and process.

The last dimension, outcome, is considered the most important and ultimate indicator of quality.[8] The bottom line of any question regarding quality of care is the resultant effect on health status. The old cliche that the operation was a success but the patient died vividly points out the difference between process and outcome.

Once we define good quality, it is necessary to translate the goal into some sort of activity. The next logical step in the process is assessment. Quality assessment refers to measuring the quality of care. Although we can, through assessment, determine the acceptability of certain aspects of care, assessment does nothing to improve the level of care. Given that some deficiencies in the care system have been identified, we must then enter the realm of quality assurance. Quality assurance is a *set of steps taken to rectify identified deficiencies in the quality of care and to prevent these deficiencies from recurring*. The concept of assurance often poses the sticky prospects of conflict, sanctions, and legal recourse but can also be a positive educational process that enhances basic behavior in the provider system. The implications of quality assurance have made it more often spoken about than realized. A recent ADA study confirms that there is a rapidly developing technology for assessment but a rather slow, lumbering one for effecting quality assurance.[9]

NATURE OF THE PROBLEM OF QUALITY OF CARE

From an individual or collective perspective, the issue of quality assurance boils down to the availability of relevant information upon which policy decisions can be made. Unfortunately, although the health-care literature is extensive,[10] we are only beginning to develop the kinds of information sources required by the consumer, provider, and the policymaker. The problems of quality facing policymakers can be classified as those that relate to (1) technical quality of the services, (2) art of care, and (3) over- or underutilization of services. Each of these problem areas has two types of cost implications. The first concerns the impact of the problem on total program costs; the second, the costs associated with identifying and resolving the problem, that is, the quality assurance system. It is by understanding the nature of each of these problem areas and its cost implications that rational policy decisions can be developed.

Technical Quality of Services

Poor technical quality of care, for the purpose of discussion, refers to improperly performed procedures. The overhanging amalgam, the root tip that is left after the tooth is extracted, the improperly filled root canal, are examples of poor technical quality. The California Dental Association's (CDA) manual, *Quality Evaluation for Dental Care*,[11] provides a good basis for defining the technical level of specific dental services. While the CDA system was developed for a direct patient examination that can be cumbersome and expensive, some criteria developed by the CDA can be adapted for indirect use on posttreatment radiographs. Another method of identifying problems in the technical quality of care is the use of tracers on computer-generated patient profiles.[12] This approach uses treatment patterns such as redos or extractions of recently restored teeth.

Thus, the technology for identifying poor technical care is developing; however, several nagging questions remain. Presently, we do not fully understand the relationship between what the profession considers poor treatment and the dental health of the patient. Certainly most clinicians are familiar with the retained root tip that remains asymptomatic in the patient's jaw. We would all agree that leaving a root tip after an extraction is poor technical care; however, in some cases the effects on the health of the patient are negligible. On the other hand, poorly adapted crowns have resulted in loss of the tooth from caries or periodontal disease.

The costs associated with these two examples of poor technical care are considerably different. In the first instance, the imposition of quality assurance would add cost but have little immediate effect on health; on the other hand, it could have an indirect effect of making the practitioner aware of his unacceptable technique. In the second case, the effect is both direct and indirect. The rectification of the poor care will save additional charges that result from the deterioration of the dentition, as well as making the practitioner aware of his inadequate performance. The decision to impose a quality-assurance system to ensure the technical quality of care is a function of (1) the extent to which unacceptable care is prevalent, (2) the effects of un-acceptable care on the dental health of the population, (3) the costs of implementing a quality-assurance system, and (4) its ability to re-solve the problem of technical quality.

Unfortunately, very few studies have addressed the extent of the problem of technical quality of care. One that does is by Gordon et al. In their report *Computer Applications for Dental Quality Assur-ance*,[13] they examined 646 patients and found that 92 percent of 11,003 restorative procedures were acceptable. Only 5 percent were considered of such poor quality that they needed to be replaced im-mediately. If, in fact, the general level of quality is so high, one might question the necessity of quality assurance that focuses on the tech-nical quality of care; however, whether these data reflect general con-ditions is still open to debate.

Art of Care

Whereas effort is being placed on developing a technology for assessing the technical level of care, the art-of-care assessment is only beginning. Without good indicators for art-of-care assessment, we are hampered in our ability to develop policies that would promote this important dimension of quality. Patient-satisfaction surveys, compli-ance with treatment regimes, and preventive home-care procedures are examples of the types of activities that reflect the art of care.[14] Separating the responsibility of the provider from that of the patient is extremely difficult. The provider's responsibility is to provide the information, training, and motivation. But to what extent can a quality-assurance system realistically get involved with this type of provider-patient interaction? The complexity of this area of assess-ment is matched by its potential benefit to dental health.

Overtreatment and Undertreatment

The next two problem areas concern utilization of services. Up to this point, we were assuming that the prescription of treatment was correct but the execution was faulty. Presently we are concerned with under- and overtreatment, where the provider does not adequately assess the patient's needs.

Let's examine the problem of undertreatment. Certainly part of the problem of undertreatment resides in consumer attitudes and perceptions. According to the HANES survey, 64 percent of the pop-ulation requires dental treatment of one or more types.[15] In a 1978 report, approximately 30 percent of people twenty-five to forty-four years old in the United States have not seen a dentist in two or more years. This statistic increases to 62 percent for the sixty-five-year-olds and over. The average number of visits per person in that year was 1.6.[16]

C. W. Douglass, in his review of utilization studies, also points out that, although more people may have access to dental care, it is clear that a large portion of the population is underutilizing.[17] In this chapter, since we are limiting the concept of utilization to those who receive dental care, underutilization would require a quality-assurance system to identify additional or more complex services for those persons. Quality assurance would thus work contrary to cost containment, since missed diagnoses could very likely result in additional, more complex, and often more expensive treatment. On the other hand, some view overtreatment as the major problem facing the dental patient.[18] Overtreatment consists of providing care when care is not necessary and also opting for expensive, complex care when simpler, less costly services would be reasonable. Quality assurance in these cases would limit service and reinforce cost containment. Thus the policymaker must consider that quality assurance is a double-edged sword which may either significantly increase or, to some degree, contain cost.

Types of Quality-Assurance Activities

Systems have been developed to address the problems of quality. These consist of combinations of review steps that examine claims, patients, or practices. The Research Triangle Institute in 1975[19] compared quality assurance (QA) activities among three types of third-party insurance carriers. The analysis showed that, although the Deltas, the Blue Cross/Blue Shield organization, and the commercial companies varied in specific approaches, QA activities revolved around the areas of single-claims review, aggregate-claims review, and non-claims-related activities. The components of quality-assurance systems have been discussed by Hillsman and are presented here so that the reader may gain some insight into the typical components of quality-assurance systems.[20] Although we recognize that there may be a divergence of opinion on these definitions, we consider them sufficiently inclusive and uncontroversial to be used here.

Nonpeer refers to a specially trained nondentist, usually a dental assistant, who takes part in the review process. These individuals can review claims forms, perform abstracting of dental records, etc. They represent the first noncomputer review that a claim receives. They do not usually make final decisions regarding the quality of care, but can identify and refer claims to a dental consultant for adjudication.

Peer refers to a graduate dentist who makes decisions regarding the quality of care. A frequently used peer is a dental consultant who may be employed either by a third party or under contract. These individuals may examine patients, conduct practice audits, review cases, etc. They represent the quality standards of the third-party organization and make decisions regarding the appropriateness of treatment, technical quality, adequacy of performance, etc. They will often resolve conflicts directly with the providers.

Peer Review Committee refers to a professionally sponsored and operated system for adjudication of disagreements relating to fees, plan reimbursements, or quality of care. This form of review is different from the dental consultant because the committee represents the profession. Peer review by committee is usually resorted to when the provider or patient cannot resolve the problem through the dental consultant.

Direct Clinical Assessment refers to patient examination requiring the patient's presence and time as well as radiographs, patient records, claims information, etc. The direct clinical exam can be performed pre- or posttreatment to authorize treatment or to determine the appropriateness or quality of the care. The dental consultant, a representative of the peer review committee, or a member of the state dental board can perform the assessment.

Indirect Patient Assessment refers to the review of patient data without requiring the patient's presence. The focus is on an individual patient and information such as patient records, radiographs, claims forms, and study models may be used in this review. Thse data may be reviewed initially by a non-peer and then by a dental consultant, if necessary.

Practice Profile refers to indirect data collected on an individual dental practice and used to identify its patterns of care. The information is generally derived from posttreatment claims forms. The practice profiles are reviewed by the dental consultant and those with aberrant patterns are selected for further investigation either through a statistical approach or through the use of standards defining appropriate types of care.

Patient Profile refers to indirect data, collected on an individual patient and usually derived from historical claims data treatment records, relating to the distribution of services provided under a program. Patient profiles, often compiled by computers, may be used to identify patients receiving specific services (e.g., dentures) or to identify seemingly inappropriate patterns of care. These profiles can be used to identify potential instances of low-quality care but do not represent the final step of quality assurance.

Practice Audit refers to a direct assessment of a practice by reviewing patient records, radiographs, and facilities. A dental consultant conducts this review on site (a nonpeer can be involved in some abstracting of information). The review focuses on the practice and the nature of the care it provides.

Sanctions refers to steps taken by the program, peer review, or state boards to require restitution from providers for inappropriate or inadequate care. Sanctions include substitution of services, nonpayment of claims, withdrawal of payment, or elimination from the program, and could extend to loss of license. The issuing of sanctions is intended to change the behavior of practitioners directly by its imposition and indirectly by setting examples.

The combination of various review steps and the interactions of components as described above provide the framework for quality-assurance systems.

INSTITUTIONAL ENVIRONMENT FOR QUALITY ASSURANCE

Basic to our discussion of quality-assurance systems and cost containment are the institutional circumstances present in the dental system that effect quality-assurance activities. Institutional entities have two dimensions by which they can be classified. The first is whether the institution is public or private and the second is related to whether it is a financial or professional entity. Clearly, dental societies represent private, professional institutions, whereas commercial insurance companies are private financial institutions. Even though there is some overlap—California Dental Services corporation is a private financial institution that does have close ties with professional societies; similarly dental practice is a private professional entity with a fiscal orientation—this method of classification enables us to examine the present and potential role for quality assurance in terms of its impact on the dental system.

The public sector consists of federal, state, and local agencies that play a financial or professional role. For example, Medicaid

administration is a publicly financed program that can affect the dental-care system in quality and cost on state and local levels.[21] The
public sector's financial role in dentistry represents a small and perhaps decreasing proportion of the total dental expenditures.

The private sector financial institutions consist of (1) commerical
insurance companies, (2) dental service corporations, (3) Blue Cross/
Blue Shield, (4) prepaid capitation plans, and (5) the diffuse group
of out-of-pocket payers. The last and least organized entity accounts
for the largest share of expenditures, amounting to 73.0 percent in
1979. Although this percentage is still high, it has been declining at a
rapid rate owing to increasing share of expenditures by third-party
private entities. In 1979, private third parties accounted for 23 percent of dental expenditures, whereas as recently as 1970 they accounted for only 5.1 percent.

The dramatic increase in the role of third parties represents an
impact by financial institutions that has been responsible for much
of the interest and activity regarding quality assurance and cost containment. Within these private financial institutions, the commercial
insurance companies account for 67 percent of the 1976 total third-
party expenditures, with Delta Dental plans accounting for 17.7 percent and Blue Cross/Blue Shield for 11 percent. The remaining 4.3
percent is spread among a number of private plans including self-insured groups, HMOs, and capitation plans.[22]

The vast majority of private financial institutions are based on a
fee-for-service method of remuneration. The small share associated
with capitation financing is growing quite rapidly in several parts of
the country. Either method of payment has to some degree used
various methods and opportunities for quality assurance. Thus, in
viewing the public and private financial institutions, the activity and
potential is predominantly found in private third-party programs.

The professional orientation, like the financial, is also found in
private and public sectors. The American Dental Association (ADA)
with its constituent societies is a major private professional institutional entity that has had an effect on the potential for quality assurance. The ADA position regarding participation in peer review through
a Professional Standards Review Organization (PSRO) is expressed
by the following position statement: "The Association readily ac-
knowledges its responsibility for dental peer review, both in private
and in public health programs. The Association believes that unless
dentists are involved in the planning and administration of PSROs, a
sound system for reviewing dental care will not likely develop."[23]

The ADA's willingness to participate in peer-review activity is confirmed by its establishment of component review committees for assessment of quality in prepayment programs.[24] The ADA has not taken a position on the audit of private dental offices by fiscal intermediaries.[25] The ADA has conducted research on the "state of the art" of dental quality assurance. A related organization, the American Fund for Dental Health, has, in conjunction with the W. K. Kellogg Foundation, established a National Dental Quality Assurance Advisory Committee to "stimulate, coordinate, monitor, and develop a national program of quality assurance in Dentistry." Through these professionally oriented research efforts, the nature and content of quality-assurance systems has developed.[26]

Public professional institutions perform valuable quality-control functions. First, they license practitioners, which theoretically restricts entry into the profession to those who have demonstrated knowledge and technical skill. The licensing function also extends to those organizations that conduct business within the state. For example, the Department of Corporations in California licenses prepaid health plans and specifies that a quality-of-care review system be a requirement for licensing.

Second, federal and local governmental agencies have a long history of providing dental care to special population groups (e.g., veterans, military personnel, Indians on reservations, merchant seamen, etc.). As public professional institutions, these programs have developed mechanisms for quality assurance.

Finally, the public sector supports research, which is reflected in projects supported by the National Center for Health Services Research, the Division of Dental Health, and the Bureau of Quality Assurance. These research programs are influential in evaluating and directing quality-assurance efforts and may enhance mandated government programs.

Within the dental sector, institutional circumstances influence the nature and direction of quality-assurance activities in a variety of ways. Presently, we think of private financial institutions (such as insurance companies) and private professional organizations (such as local dental societies) as being the most important and influential institutions. However, we may begin to see other entities evolve such as the professional financial bodies (franchises). In exchange for providing practitioners with an opportunity to buy into an advertising entity, franchises would possibly require a peer review system and site review.[27] They can be expected to use the existence of quality assurance to enhance the marketing of their organizations.

ECONOMIC INCENTIVES AND THE MARKET
FOR QUALITY ASSURANCE

Three basic parties are involved in the market for dental care: the first party is the patient-consumer; the second is the provider; and the third is the fiscal intermediary, either public or private.

Consumers

It is assumed that consumers purchase goods and services that are selected so that satisfaction is maximized. The constraint that an individual consumer faces is an overall budget that limits the total amount he or she can spend on all goods and services. It is useful to remember that it is not dental care per se that gives the consumer satisfaction; rather, it is the individual's concept of dental health that the consumer values. Dental care is one of several inputs into the process by which dental health is obtained (the production function). Other inputs include oral hygiene, nutrition, etc. The relevant question facing each consumer is the following: Within my budget, how much should I spend on the professional dental care that contributes to my dental health?

If one assumes that consumers are averse to risks, then reducing the uncertainty associated with the consumption of dental care will have some value to them. That is, they will be willing to pay some premium for a reduction in the uncertainty that they face in consuming dental care—whether the uncertainty is caused by fear of incorrect advice or by questioning an unknown provider's competence.[28] The relevant question is how much consumers would be willing to pay for this information, and whether this premium is as large as the extra cost associated with providing it. From economic theory, we would expect that consumers will choose to consume QA until the marginal benefit that they would get from one additional unit of QA is less than their cost in obtaining that unit.

It is important to keep in mind that these costs and benefits may be pecuniary and nonpecuniary and that both components are important. For example, as mentioned above, patients often do not have adequate information to make optimal decisions regarding dental treatment. If quality assurance can supply this type of information, it may be beneficial to consumers, depending on what it costs them. On the other hand, the patient-provider relationship is strongly institutionalized and may conflict with efforts toward quality assurance. If quality assurance appears to be a bureaucratic waste of time, or if it denies a benefit to the consumer that the provider has recommended, the consumer may resist the efforts of quality-assurance systems.

Providers

An added complexity, however, arises here. For consumers to select the "correct" amount and type of dental care (to maximize their utility), they must have some idea of the relationship between dental care and dental health. Given the technical nature of dental care, this relationship is not always obvious to consumers. Furthermore, as mentioned previously, there are several alternative treatments for a given condition. Dentistry, as a technical service, can be quite complex, and it is questionable whether consumers have the information with which to make informed choices in selecting optimal types and amounts of dental care. Since obtaining the necessary information may be expensive and time-consuming, several institutions have arisen to provide it. One very important institution is the patient-dentist agency relationship.

Patients ask dentists to act on their behalf and select the appropriate types and amounts of dental care, given their individual dental health. The relationship has worked reasonably well but has several limitations. It should be noted that patient-consumers still face the budgeting constraints usually encountered when buying goods and services. Choosing to purchase dental care means that each consumer must forgo some other good, service, savings, or activity.

Perfect agency relationships imply that dentists know what patients need and want and clearly understand the relationship between process and outcome. Each of these assumptions may be questioned. Another problem is that trusting in patient-doctor relationships to provide patients with optimal information assumes that the patients and dentists have the same interests. It is useful to consider the economic incentives that influence the behavior of dentists.

We begin with the assumption that dentists produce levels of quality and amounts of care that they hope will maximize their profits. There are, of course, other motivations that influence the behavior of dentists (such as the satisfaction they receive from performing high-quality work). But for our purposes, it is assumed that dentists are motivated primarily by profit maximization. In this situation, conflicting forces might cause providers to choose other than technically ideal types of care.

In dentistry, there are often alternative treatments appropriate for the same dental condition. Since high-quality dental care can require more resources and therefore cost more, some consumers might prefer to purchase lower-quality dental care, given a lower price, just as other consumers in other settings might choose Subarus rather than Mercedes. An example in dentistry is the choice between a gold onlay and a three-surface amalgam. While the former might be considered superior (in terms of durability), the latter is far less expensive and can be considered a substitute. From the point of view of dentists, the gold treatment might be preferable (assuming fee-for-service) if it were more profitable. Each consumer has a choice too—whether the marginal improvement in dental health resulting from the gold treatment is worth the difference in price.

There is, moreover, the question of the agency relationship. If consumers are given the information about the probable outcomes associated with each type of treatment, product differentiation is possible and the market will operate efficiently in the selection of quality levels. But we cannot always be assured that the incentives under which providers operate are incentives to convey the best available information (i.e., that agency relationships are complete). This issue is crucial in deciding the appropriate role of quality assurance.

Let us assume for now that product differentiation occurs, that utilization levels are correct, and that some consumers select gold onlays while others opt for silver fillings. Within each type of treatment there is a range of quality variation owing to a number of factors. While care is being delivered, dentists might remove excessive tooth structure, or delivery might be inadequate, and any of a number of other factors might affect the outcomes of treatment. Reducing these uncertainties increases the value of dental care to consumers. Quality assurance may be used to reduce the variations in outcome that arise during the selected treatments. That is, given that an individual consumer has opted for, say, the three-surface amalgam, he or she would like to be reasonably sure that the amalgam is a good one. To ensure that the technical quality of care is up to some chosen level, preauthorization claims review, licensure, practice audits, and other quality-assurance systems can be employed. There is, of course, a random component of outcome inherent in the practice of dentistry. That is, no matter how good the provider is, there is a nonzero probability that a procedure will fail. To reduce this uncertainty, research funding is probably more appropriate than quality assurance.

Thus, providers may benefit or lose from QA. If dentists do good work, reinforced by QA, their reputations and patient-provider relationship will be strengthened. (Of course, one does observe poor dentists who maintain good reputations by compensating for technical inadequacy with superb chairside manners and vice versa. This seeming paradox is explained by remembering that there are other components to quality of care than just technical treatment, and perspectives on what constitutes good quality care differ among individuals, providers, third parties, etc.) In addition, providers will have incentives to monitor care. An individual provider's profit levels should respond to a growing reputation and patient satisfaction. However, reputation, independence, and the agency relationship itself may be threatened by the perceived intrusion into a provider's domain. A provider may gain in receiving information on how to provide better dental care. But this may be threatening to the provider, and he or she may question whether the evaluators are in a position to pass judgment.

Fiscal Intermediaries

Thus far we have been describing how various levels of quality might be chosen and how variations in quality within alternative treatments might arise. It has also been suggested that quality assurance might have a role to play in determining the "correct" utilization level of treatment and reducing variations in technical quality. There are several additional important questions in analyzing the role of quality assurance. First, does the private market provide optimal quality assurance? Second, if not, is there reason for government intervention?

The increasing role of third-party payment has greatly affected the market for dental care and the potential for quality assurance. Because insurance lowers the out-of-pocket cost of dental care at the time of delivery, there is a substitution effect and people demand more care. This has been widely discussed in the literature.[29] In addition, upgrading to higher levels of quality also takes place. Provisions of insurance programs affect the behavior of dentists as well as consumers. In a minimally funded benefit program offering high coinsurance and deductibles, providers might respond to low reimbursement rates by limiting involvement or overprescribing patient care to obtain more acceptable rates of return. In a well-funded program, there is strong incentive for overtreatment.

Insurance also creates a wedge between the prices paid by consumers and those received by dentists. When an individual patient selects among treatments and providers decide whether the perceived difference in quality is worth the difference in price, the patient makes the calculation using the out-of-pocket cost. However, the actual cost to society is the gross cost. Thus, this undervaluation leads to inefficient overconsumption of services or overtreatment.

At the same time, however, third-party indemnity programs have incentives to contain costs to remain competitive in their insurance marketplace. If quality assurance reinforces cost containment, third parties will favor it. Otherwise, they may not. In addition to this consideration, the demonstration of an effective quality-assurance system might tend to make any type of prepaid program more attractive from a marketing standpoint.

QUALITY-ASSURANCE SYSTEMS: A CLOSER LOOK

As we have pointed out, quality assurance consists of a series of review steps that influence the quality of care and the costs associated with each state of review. Some QA systems process claims; others, patients; and still others, dental practices. To illustrate the relationship between costs and quality-assurance systems, we have selected the preauthorization of claims. Table 1 is a schematic representation of the various steps associated with this common type of quality-assurance system.[30] The appendix gives more detail about the models developed by the authors and illustrates their operation with numerical examples.

The claims-review process has two concerns: administrative and professional decisions. Most of the administrative decisions associated with the claims-review process involve a determination of benefits: that is, whether the service requested is covered under the particular plan. These decisions, while effecting cost containment, are not a quality-assurance activity. The vast majority of decisions made by third parties are of this type.

The decisions requiring professional judgment have implications for quality assurance. In these instances, the judgments concern the appropriateness of care sought on the preauthorization claims requests. For example, a dentist may request an extraction of a first molar to be replaced by a three-unit bridge. A dental consultant might review the case and authorize an endodontic procedure and a crown. This example represents a decision on the appropriateness of care for services covered by the plan. Presently, most programs restrict their review process to the determination of benefits rather than the difficult area of appropriateness of care. Nevertheless, the potential exists for the use of the preauthorization mechanism as part of a quality-assurance system.

In a typical preauthorization system, all claims over $100 might first be screened by a nonpeer. In cases where the nonpeer has questions about the appropriateness of the work proposed, a dental consultant performs an indirect review of the claim (using radiographs but not requiring the patient's presence). This is the first stage at which quality assurance can influence the care delivered. If the

Table 1. A Preauthorization Claims Review Process Based on Dollar Amount
(with direct patient examination by dental consultant)

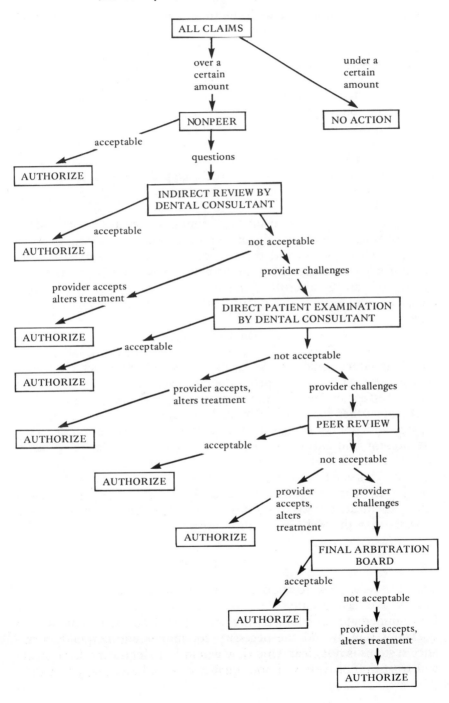

consultant does not agree with the treatment plan of the provider, he or she will propose an alternative.

At this point, the original provider may accept the consultant's directive, in which case the treatment would be approved; or the dentist may challenge the consultant's findings to a higher level of review — a direct examination by the consultant. The consultant (not necessarily the same one) would then perform a direct patient exam and may either approve or suggest modifications to the preauthorization-request. The provider has the same options available: to modify the claim or challenge it to a higher review step. The review sequence may go on to a peer-review committee (representing the profession) and a final arbitration board (whose decisions are considered final and binding).

As the model developed in the appendix illustrates, costs and impacts of quality assurance depend on the population at risk, provider and patient requests, and the particular type of quality assurance being used. Of course, of primary concern is what happens to the quality of care as a result of quality assurance. If quality-assurance decisions are correct, the quality of care will be enhanced in two major ways. First, as a result of better care, the dental-health status of patients should improve (in Donabedian's terms, improving the process of care improves the outcome of care). Second, quality assurance is an educational process for providers and, if correct, gives them information on how to improve the quality of work. This will have a positive effect in the present and future if providers heed the advice.

On the other hand, if an individual quality-assurance decision is wrong, and poorer care is delivered, these benefits become costs in the present and future. Moreover, the patient-provider relationship has been intruded upon, which may hurt the art-of-care dimension of quality. This latter effect will occur whether the quality-assurance decision is right or wrong. Thus a key question is whether intrusions into patient-dentist relationships are justified by the expected improvement in the technical quality of care.

CONCLUSIONS

Our discussion has focused on the interaction between costs and quality. We have isolated the problems of quality and seen that they have immediate and long-term effects on costs. Many unanswered questions remain and the necessity for implementing quality-assurance systems is not clear. One view would be to let the market operate and trust that providers of poor-quality care will eventually lose their patients, while providers who serve the needs of their patients will prosper. Malpractice litigation is also pointed to as a mechanism for controlling quality. Yet, it is reasonable to assume that most concerned providers and consumers do not feel that market forces or malpractice mechanisms are adequate QA safeguards.

The profession has, through its peer-review committees, acted as a safety valve to arbitrate conflicts between consumers and providers; whatever one's opinion of the effectiveness of peer-review activities, they do not provide a system of quality assurance. Much talk concerns the role of third parties in this area. However, we do not have a great deal of evidence that third parties are anxious to attack the problems of quality. What about consumers? Are consumers, either as individuals or collectively, interested in quality assurance? Generally there is lip service paid to quality by managers of union and management health-care financial systems, but are they willing to put up the dollars or take the heat? The answer is usually no.

The government has taken some interest in quality assurance. PSROs are an example of federal legislation that uses external review of the appropriateness of hospital use, but the relative emphasis on quality vs. cost containment in this effort has been the source of much confusion.[31] In addition, there is a growing laissez-faire attitude among government officials to let the dental market operate with a minimum of government intervention. The small amount of public funding for dental care will probably be reduced, resulting in a smaller role for the federal government in quality assurance. At the state level, boards of dental examiners, according to Milgrom, show a promising trend toward "moving away from a punitive or disciplinary view of regulation to a position where quality assurance is viewed as an ongoing responsibility."[32] Another potential model for quality assurance at the state level is found in the role of the Department of Corporations of the State of California which licenses health-care service plans.[33] The law requires internal quality-review systems for each prepaid dental plan. This type of legislation sees quality-assurance systems as an integral part of the operation of prepaid dental-care programs. The extent to which this mandate will be exercised remains to be seen. The present reality seems to be that quality assurance is hovering, but it is finding it rather difficult to locate a safe place to land.

The need for quality-assurance systems will become more and more apparent if present trends continue. The paramount problem of quality is related to the appropriateness of care rather than to technical adequacy. With the growing dental-insurance industry, primarily based on fee-for-service reimbursement, with increased competition among dentists for patients, with decline in caries and edentulism, with increased risk of periodontal disease, and with rising costs of establishing and operating a dental practice, dentists will face growing economic pressures to maximize the return on each patient. This generally means providing as many high-priced services as possible. If we agree "that many expensive dental services have small marginal effects on oral health,"[34] then the need for and challenge of quality-assurance systems is quite clear. The paradox is that the major third-party programs have countered increased costs by changing benefit structures and imposing annual maximums and deductibles; but limiting utilization by patients does not represent a real effort to deal with the overutilization issue.[35]

Furthermore, even those programs that do preauthorize treatment are not in a strong position to affect overuse. In all cases, there is a dollar limit above which a claim requires preauthorization. The potential for abuse is quite wide when one considers the possibility that a provider can create the condition below the preauthorization limit that would justify its authorization above the limit. For example, a dentist could extract several teeth and request payment without review because the claim was below the $100 preauthorization level. Then the provider could request several hundred dollars to replace these teeth, which would be approved because the replacements are required. However, the original decision to remove the teeth might not have been correct. Thus, the claims services preauthorization approach can be circumvented by dentists who wish to do so. Therefore, quality-assurance systems based on claims considerations alone hold only minimal potential for coping with and rectifying the overuse problem. Thus, cost containment is managed primarily by design of benefit structure and determination of benefits.

The Future of Quality Assurance

The present uncertainty will clear somewhat as the information and technology associated with quality develops. We can hope that the primary focus of quality assurance will be on individual providers and consumers. The provider's awareness of quality-assessment procedures will encourage the institution of formal approaches in the practice. Although these efforts may add costs initially, the long-term effects may be increased viability of the practice. As consumers learn to utilize information either collectively or as individuals, they will become a greater part of the decision-making process. Whether this information takes the form of shoppers' guides,[36] advertising, popular literature,[37] or advice from dentists, it will open the way for improved quality of care.

Others will participate at a different level. The marketing of prepaid plans will continue; and we can hope that, as the marketplace settles, purchasers will give more consideration to quality assurance. Outside opinions from dental faculty and other consultant groups will be necessary to provide the expertise for purchasing groups. Dental education will also have to emphasize a broader concept of quality, including the teaching of evaluation techniques. The profession will have to continue its leadership in research and training so that its membership understands and accepts its responsibility. The government, first at the state level, will view its licensure role as a continuing one, perhaps involving certification of practices. At the federal level, we can hope for support of research, development, and training programs devoted to quality assurance. But it is unlikely that, without a national dental health insurance program, we can expect federal regulation concerning dental-care quality assurance.

It would simplify matters if myriad issues touched upon in this paper could be synthesized into a common thread. Unfortunately, uncertainties prevail and much must be done to clear the issues that surround quality assurance. Perhaps the two opposing points of view boil down to the following: (1) market forces will naturally serve as a quality-assurance system, and (2) it is in the best interest of consumers and providers to set up external review systems to monitor and influence the quality of care produced by the system. There are costs, problems, and risks involved in either position. The challenge of the next decade will be to find, with initiative and creativity, a path that simultaneously serves the needs of consumers and providers.

Appendix: A Model Estimating Costs of Quality Assurance

The concepts of quality assurance and their relationship to costs are not easily understood. In the face of limited data, we present a model that illustrates some of the relationships between costs and quality assurance. It should be noted that the numbers used in the following examples are hypothetical and are for illustration only, although they are based on real-world estimates. It is believed that these estimates are internally consistent and can reasonably illustrate how quality-assurance systems function. We have chosen preauthorization review for extensive illustration. The model presented here allows us to examine relationships among various sets of input parameters and outputs (direct cost of operating quality assurance, distribution of services, impact of quality assurance, etc.) This model was developed by the authors to examine the administrative costs of various QA systems for the dental component of any national health-insurance legislation.[38] (This model has been made into a computer program that simulates the interactions which might take place among program benefits, administrative costs, total program costs, and the distribution of dental services requested. HRA contract No. 231-77-0076).

The model operates on a set of equations that contain the following three components: *requests* made in a program, a *linking generator*, and the *quality-assurance system*. The model predicts a distribution in terms of the costs and quantities of dental services for nine major service categories. The inputs to the model are the size of eligible population, population utilization rate, average number of services per user, and the percentage distribution of various categories of services. Table 2 presents these inputs for two programs with different

Table 2. Input Parameters and Results of Quality-Assurance Model

	High-Level Program 1	Low-Level Program 2
Input Parameters		
Population	10,000.0	10,000.0
Utilization rate	60.0%	60.0%
Services per user	5.5	5.5
Diagnostic	21.3	40.6
Preventive	17.5	34.7
Operative	15.4	16.5
Crown and bridge	39.9	2.0
Prosthetics	3.0	0.5
Oral surgery	2.2	2.4
Endodontics	0.2	0.9
Periodontics	0.5	2.5
Orthodontics	0.0	0.0
Results		
Diag-cost	$ 1,054.	$ 2,010.
No. of services	7,029.	13,398.
Prev-cost	$ 1,039.	$ 2,061.
No. of services	5,775.	11,451.
Oper-cost	$ 1,016.	$ 1,089.
No. of services	5,082.	5,445.
C & b-cost	$ 28,243.	$ 1,416.
No. of services	13,167.	660.
Pros-cost	$ 2,772.	$ 462.
No. of services	990.	165.
O.S.-cost	$ 152.	$ 166.
No. of services	726.	792.
Endo-cost	$ 78.	$ 350.
No. of services	66.	297.
Perio-cost	$ 87.	$ 433.
No. of services	165.	825.
Ortho-cost	$ 0.	$ 0.
No. of services	0.	0.
Total cost	$3,444,200.	$798,700.
Total number of services	33,000.	33,033.

levels of service requests. In this example, the eligible population of 10,000 people have the same utilization rates and average number of services per user. The only difference between the two hypothetical plans is the distribution of services requested. In the high-request plan, 39.9 percent of all services are crown and bridgework, compared to only 2.0 percent in the low-request plan. The outputs from this component of the model are the number and cost of services for each service category. The average cost per eligible claim for a high level of requests is $344.42 compared to $79.87 for the low request plan.

The administrative costs related to preauthorization quality assurance and impact costs resulting from quality assurance were calculated and are presented in tables 3 and 4 under various assumptions about the request level that existed before QA review. Because, in preauthorization decisions, one of the chief concerns is whether providers are requesting appropriate levels of services, the question arises whether the requested utilization represents undertreatment, overtreatment, or appropriate treatment. In an actual quality-assurance system, of course, each preauthorization claim would be evaluated on its own merits. However, in this type of simulation, a priori expectations must be integrated into the model.

To treat each claim separately, a simple probabilistic transitional model was incorporated into the simulation. This submodel provides a framework for estimating the types of changes that a quality-assurance system might mean in terms of the distribution of services. It simulates the additions, deletions, and changes in individual categories of dental services.

High Requests

Using two different patterns of service request (high and low levels), we can examine how the preauthorization approach to QA operates in terms of costs and impacts. The high-request level represents provider responses to a dental-care program for a population of 10,000 eligibles, which includes a lot of crown and bridge requests. Table 3 gives summary information on the total number of claims, the administrative costs as a percentage of total program costs, and per-claim administrative costs. In addition, for each of the three assumptions concerning service utilization level, it shows a variety of measures of the financial impact that QA might have.

In the middle of table 3, the number of claims reaching each review step and the administrative costs associated with each are presented. The review process for the high-request pattern resolves all claims by the fourth step, which involves a direct patient exam by a dental consultant.

The impact costs vary according to whether there are over-, under-, or appropriate service utilization levels being requested. If utilization levels are appropriate, quality assurance will not affect the number or distribution of services provided. Therefore, impact costs will be zero and quality assurance will be a financial drain on the program. On the other hand, if there is overutilization and quality assurance corrects it, service costs will be reduced. At the other extreme, if under the high-request program, users were underutilizing services and if quality assurance corrected the program, there would be additional service costs.

Again, we wish to emphasize that the numerical results are entirely dependent upon the assumptions inherent in the choice of input parameters and on assumptions inherent in the simulation model itself. Infinite variations on these assumptions are possible. By entering two very different sets of input parameters, each of which is purely hypothetical but internally consistent, we have shown that the model is sensitive to the values selected.

Low Requests

The low-request program would provide primarily diagnostic and preventive care. Therefore, the costs of the entire program and average costs per claim are much lower than in the high-request program ($0.8 million versus $3.4 million and $70 versus $270 per claim respectively (see table 4). The administrative costs of QA are also much lower since the claims are much simpler, smaller, and therefore less likely to be selected for review.

The middle section of table 4 shows the progression of claims through the QA system. By comparing this with table 3, it is clear that claims are resolved earlier in the low-request program. For example, in the high-request program, only 52 percent of all claims are resolved by the dollar screen. In the low-request program, 84 percent are under $100. As in the high-request program, whether quality assurance is cost-adding or cost-saving depends on the original service utilization level of providers under the program.

The comparison of these two levels of requests shows that a given quality-assurance system would react in very different ways. In the high-request example, the costs of the quality assurance system were $61,644 compared to $11,263 in the low-request program. Even though the tendency is to increase direct costs, the total effect (assuming overutilization) is a cost savings of 3.38 percent, whereas the low-request example has a limited cost savings of

Table 3. Summary Statistics for a Claims Review QA System
Applied to a High-Request Program

Cost of program $3,442,031.
Number of claims   12,744.
Cost per claim $270.09

Application of QAS 1: Claims Preauthorization System

Administrative cost $ 61,644.
Administrative cost
  as a percentage of (1)   1.79%
Administrative cost
  per claim $4.83

Description of Review Step	Number of Claims at This Step	Percentage of Claims Resolved at This Step	Administrative Costs of This Review Step
Initial dollar screen	12,744	52.1	$ 2,039.
Non-peer review	7,952.	32.5	19,562.
Indirect review by dental consultant	3,471.	14.2	30,371.
Direct exam by dental consultant	303.	1.2	9,572.
Peer review committee	0.	0.0	0.
Final arbitration board	0.	0.0	0.
		100.0	$61,544.

	Assuming Underutilization	Assuming Overutilization	Assuming Correct Utilization
Change in service costs	$111,000	−$178,000	0
Net costs	$172,544	−$116,456	$61,544
Net cost as a percentage of (1)	5.01%	−3.38%	1.79%
Net cost per claim	$13.54	−$9.14	$4.83
Cost of providing services	$3,614,575	$3,325,575	$3,503,575
Cost per claim	$283.63	$260.95	$274.92

0.42 percent. Thus the response of quality assurance can vary depending on the nature of the requests, the extent of problems encountered, and the vigilance of the quality-assurance system itself.

A Richer Model

The simulation model thus far has provided a basis for estimating the costs of quality-assurance systems for different request patterns. It has been assumed that the work requested under a specific benefit structure can be characterized as representing predominantly under-, over-, or appropriately utilized dental services. Although all claims are considered separately, all errors in utilization level are assumed to be in the same direction. In fact, under any dental program, claims have a distribution of utilization levels; that is, some overutilize, some underutilize, and some are acceptable. The benefit structure of an insurance plan affects this distribution but will not ordinarily affect all claims in the same way. In addition, while

Table 4. Summary Statistics for a Claims Review QA System
Applied to a Low-Request Program

Cost of program	$799,281.		
Number of claims	11,310.		
Cost per claim	70.67		

Application of QAS 1: Claims Preauthorization System

Administrative cost	$ 11,263.		
Administrative cost as a percentage of (1)	1.41%		
Administrative cost per claim	$1.00		

Description of Review Step	Number of Claims Resolved at This Step	Percentage of Claims Resolved at This Step	Administrative Costs of This Review Step
Initial dollar screen	11,310	84.5	$ 1,810.
Non-peer review	1,578	11.8	3,882.
Indirect review by dental consultant	449	3.3	3,929.
Direct exam by dental consultant	52	0.4	1,643.
Peer review committee	0	0.0	0.
Final arbitration board	0	0.0	0.
		100.0	$11,263.

	Assuming Underutilization	Assuming Overutilization	Assuming Correct Utilization
Change in service costs	$13,400	−$14,600	0
Net costs	$24,663	−$3,337	$11,263
Net cost as a percentage of (1)	3.09%	−0.42%	1.41%
Net cost per claim	$2.18	−$0.30	$1.00
Cost of providing services	$828,943	$795,943	$810,544
Cost per claim	$72.85	$70.38	$71.67

the model has allowed some flexibility in testing assumptions about the degree of provider compliance and the sequence of review steps, it has not explicitly incorporated assumptions about the level of technical quality being provided. Finally, although the model has allowed us to look at costs and impacts of quality assurance under various assumptions, it has not directly addressed the advisability of implementing a quality-assurance system. For this purpose, therefore, we now present a policy model that permits policymakers to explore their subjective beliefs about quality assurance.

In this section, the model is described with an example of how it might be used to decide whether quality assurance is beneficial under either of the above two request patterns. Simply put, when we consider decisions concerning the advisability of quality-assurance systems, we must account for dimensions of technical acceptability (acceptable or not acceptable), utilization level appropriateness (over-, under-, or appropriate) and accuracy of quality-assurance evaluation (correct or incorrect). This implies a 2 x 3 x 2 matrix of all possible combinations. Table 5 presents a probability matrix that links patterns of utilization with technical quality and accuracy of quality-assurance systems. Policymakers can "plug in" their own probabilities based on everything from objective information to subjective hunches.

A set of hypothetical values has been given for illustration in this table. Multiplying these three types of probabilities (one for each dimension), we obtain the probability distribution of a set of claims. Using these values, we can analyze the implications of quality assurance from the standpoint of the multiplicity of decisions that can occur. For example, in our high-request level, the average claim has a value of $270 (see table 3). Of the 12,744 claims, 48.7 percent (6,206) will be evaluated correctly by the quality-assurance system in terms of utilization and the provision of good-quality care. In 4.5 percent of 573 claims, we assume that the quality-assurance system will correctly assess that the utilization is acceptable but that the resultant technical quality will be poor. Finally, we assume that the quality-assurance system will correctly identify 1.4 percent of 178 claims as overutilizing *and* being liable to produce poor technical care. This last situation represents the area where quality assurance will be most productive because it will not only control for overutilization but will also prevent the additional liability of these unnecessary procedures being technically unacceptable. With high requests, we assume that correct quality-assurance decisions (where changes are necessary) would account for 3,352 claims. The majority of the changes would be in the direction of reducing costs. From this point of view, the policymaker would be inclined to favor implementation of quality assurance.

The previous discussion did not take into account the affect of any incorrect decisions made by quality assurance. The dominant impact of incorrect decisions occurs where quality assurance judges that the claims are correct when in fact there are problems of quality. In our example, 2,065 claims (worth $557,000) are assumed to be incorrectly judged as having acceptable quality when the claims are indeed associated with problems of poor quality. These errors would tend to work against containing costs. Also, approximately 1,121 claims (worth $303,000) are assumed to be identified as having problems of poor quality, when in fact the quality was acceptable. This represents a sticky problem in that there is likely to be considerable justified resistance from providers and consumers. Therefore, it is in the interest of the policymaker to minimize these errors without imposing limitations that would negate the function of the quality-assurance system. A decision to make the quality-assurance system more accurate would require more resources and would add administrative costs to the system. The decision whether quality assurance should be implemented will depend on the distribution of probabilities (representing different situations) in table 5 and on the costs and benefits associated with each situation. The policymaker must assign a dollar value per claim to the costs or benefits in each cell in table 5. When these values are mutliplied by the number of claims in each cell and summed, an overall decision on the advisability of quality assurance of this type can be made.

Table 5. Matrix of Components Entering into Quality-Assurance Decisions

	Overutilization (.213)		Underutilization (.077)		Appropriate Utilization (.710)	
	Technically acceptable (.915)	Technically not acceptable (.085)	Technically acceptable (.915)	Technically not acceptable (.085)	Technically acceptable (.915)	Technically not acceptable (.085)
QA Correct (.75)	(.915 x .213 x .75) .146	(.085 x .213 x .75) .014	(.915 x .077 x .75) .053	(.085 x .077 x .75) .005	(.915 x .710 x .75) .487	(.085 x .710 x .75) .045
QA Incorrect (.25)	(.915 x .213 x .25) .049	(.085 x .213 x .25) .004	(.915 x .077 x .25) .018	(.085 x .077 x .25) .002	(.915 x .710 x .25) .162	(.085 x .710 x .25) .015

Notes

1. Roger Irving Lee and Lewis Webster Jones. *The Fundamentals of Good Medical Care*, Publication of the Committee on Costs of Medical Care, No. 22, Chicago, 1933.

2. Robert Henry Brook, Kathleen Nies Williams, and Allyson Davies Avery, "Quality Assurance Today and Tomorrow: Forecast for the Future," *Annals of Internal Medicine* 85, (6), 1976: 809-817.

3. Avedis Donabedian. *The Definition of Quality and Approaches to Its Assessment, Exploration in Quality Assessment and Monitoring*. Vol. 1. (Ann Arbor, Michigan: Health Administration Press, 1980.)

4. Robert Henry Brook, Kathleen Nies Williams, and Allyson Davies Avery. "Quality Assurance in the 20th Century: Will It Lead to Improved Health in the 21st?" in *Quality Assurance in Health Care*, ed. Richard Harrison Egdahl and Paul M. Gertman. (Germantown, Maryland: Aspen Systems Corporation, 1976), pp. 3-29.

5. California Dental Association. *Quality Evaluation for Dental Care, Guidelines for the Assessment of Clinical Quality and Professional Performance and the Standards for Program Design to Assure the Quality of Care of the California Dental Association*. (Los Angeles: California Dental Association, 1976.)

6. Howard L. Bailit et al. "Quality of Dental Care: Development of Standards," *Journal of the American Dental Association* 89, (4), October, 1974:842-853.

7. Aveais Donabedian, "Evaluating the Quality of Medical Care," *Milbank Memorial Fund Quarterly* 44, 1966:166-206.

8. Marvin Marcus, Jay A. Gershen, Alma L. Koch. *Development of Oral Health Status Measures for Quality Assurance*. UCLA School of Dentistry, National Dental Quality Assurance Program, American Fund for Dental Health, W. K. Kellogg Foundation, Final Report, 1980.

9. American Dental Association. *Quality Assurance in Dentistry*. Washington, D.C.: Department of Health, Education, and Welfare, Contract No. 240-76-0066, 1978.

10. Paul T. Sanazaro. "Quality Assessment and Quality Assurance in Medical Care," *Annual Review of Public Health*, 1,1980:37-68.

11. California Dental Association, *Quality Evaluation for Dental Care*.

12. Ronald G. DeVincenzi and Gunnar Ryge. "Using Computer Technology for Screening in Dental Quality Assurance," *California Dental Association Journal* 7, (10), 1979:31-45.

13. Daniel F. Gordon. *California Foundation for Dental Health. Computer Applications for Dental Quality Assurance*. American Fund for Dental Health (Chicago) and W. K. Kellogg Foundation (Michigan), Final Report, May, 1979.

14. LuAnn Aday, Ronald Anderson and Gretchen Fleming. *Health Care in the U.S. Equitable for Whom?* (Beverly Hills, Ca: Sage Publications, Inc., 1980), pp. 143-163.

15. *Basic Data on Dental Examination Findings of Persons 1-74 Years, United States, 1971-1974*. Hyatsville, Maryland: U.S. Department of Health, Education, and Welfare, Publication No. (PHS) 79-1662, May, 1979.

16. *Current Estimates from the Health Interview Survey: United States, 1978*. Hyatsville, Maryland: U.S. Department of Health, Education, and Welfare, Publication No. (PHS) 80-1551, November 1979, pp. 4-29.

17. Chester W. Douglass and K. O. Cole. "Utilization of Dental Services in the United States," *Journal of Dental Education* 43, (4), 1979:223-238.

18. Jay W. Friedman. "PSRO's in Dentistry," *American Journal of Public Health* 65, (12), 1975:1298-1303.

19. Research Triangle Institute. *A Study of Dental Health Related and Process Outcome Associated with Pre-Paid Dental Care*. Department of Health, Education, and Welfare, 231-76-0098, March 1977.

20. Joe T. Hillsman. "Quality Assurance in Dentistry: A Perspective," *Journal of the American Dental Association* 97, (5), November, 1978:787-790.

21. Lowell E. Bellin and Florence Kaviler. "Policing Publicly Funded Health Care for Poor Quality, Over Utilization and Fraud – New York City Medicaid Experience," *American Journal of Public Health* 60, May 1970:811 pp.

22. Marjorie Smith Carroll. "Private Health Insurance Plans in 1976: An Evaluation," *Social Security Bulletin*, 41, (9), September, 1978:3-16.

23. American Dental Association. *Dentistry in Health Legislation Policies and Positions*, Aug. 1977:p. 19.

24. American Dental Association. *Policies on Dental Care Program*. Council on Dental Care Programs, January, 1979:25.

25. *Ibid.*, p. 23.

26. National Dental Quality Assurance Advisory Committee of the American Fund for Dental Health. *Executive Summary of Dental Quality Assurance Workshop*. W. K. Kellogg Foundation/American Fund for Dental Health, June, 1979.

27. Chris S. Corby. "The Birth of Franchise Dentistry," *Dental Economics*, May 1979: 53-55.

28. Charles E. Phelps. "Benefit/Cost Analysis of Quality Assurance Programs," in *Quality Assurance in Health Care*, ed. Ralph Harrison Egdahl and Paul M. Gertman. (Germantown, Maryland: Aspen Systems Corporation, 1976), pp. 289-329.

29. Willard G. Manning and Charles E. Phelps. *Dental Care Demand: Point Estimates and Implications for National Health Insurance* (Santa Monica, Ca. The Rand Corporation, R-2157-HEW, March, 1978); Jesse S. Hixon and Nina Mocnick. *The Aggregate Supplies and Demands of Physician and Dental Services. The Target Income Hypothesis and Related Issues in Health Manpower Policy*; Paul J. Feldstein. *Financing Dental Care: An Economic Analysis*. (Lexington, Ma: D.C. Heath and Co., 1973); Charles Upton and William Silverman. "The Demand for Dental Services," *Journal of Human Resources* 7, (2), 1972:250-261.

30. Susan T. Reisine and Howard Bailit. "History and Organization of Pretreatment Review, a Dental Utilization Review System," *Public Health Reports* 95, (3), 1980:282-290.

31. Lowell E. Bellin. "PSRO: Quality Control? or Gimmickery?" *Medical Care* 12, 1974:1012-1018; Clark C. Havighurst and James F. Blumstein. "Coping with Quality/Cost Tradeoffs in Medical Care: the Role of PSRO's," *Northwestern Law Review* 70, 1975:6-68; Office of Planning, Evaluation, and Legislation. *HSA vs DHEW: Professional Standards Review Organizations: Program Evaluation*. Volume I, Washington, D.C. U.S. Dept. of HEW, 1978.

32. Peter Milgrom. *Regulation and the Quality of Dental Care*. (Germantown, Md; Aspen System Corporation, 1978), pp. 53-54.

33. Knox Keene Health Care Service Plans Act of 1975. Title 10, Articles 7, 8, 10.

34. John W. Knutson. "Controlling the Cost of Dental Health Care Insurance," *American Journal of Public Health* 69, (7), July 1979:647-648.

35. Israel L. Praiss et al. "Changing Patterns and Implications for Cost and Quality of Dental Care," *Inquiry* 16, (2), Summer 1979:131-140.

36. Herbert S. Denenberg. *A Shopper's Guide to Dentistry: Thirty-Two Rules for Selecting the Dentist and Obtaining Good Dental Care with Representative Dental Fees Changes in Pennsylvania*. (Harrisburg, Pa: Pennsylvania Insurance Department, February, 1973.)

37. Paul Revere. *Dentistry and Its Victims*. (New York: St. Martin's Press, 1970.)

38. Marvin Marcus, Max H. Schoen, Samuel J. Tobin, Describe and Document the Cost of Quality Assurance Mechanisms in National Health Insurance Programs. Final Report, DHEW Contract No. 231-77-0076, April 1980.

7

Summary and Research Suggestions

Robert T. Kudrle and Lawrence Meskin

As any reader of this book quickly recognizes, there are not only different concepts of "cost" but varying opinions on the most promising areas for cost reduction in dental care. Many of the differences among the authors in the weight they place on different factors result directly from their different assignments. Yet there remains disagreement—or at least different emphasis—among several of the chapters on such issues as the critical barriers to more effective employment of auxiliaries, the potential of outside capital and management to encourage lower production costs, the present efficiency of the dental-care system, the ability of dentists to control their incomes, and the future course of incomes in dentistry.

The editors do not presume to reconcile these differing points of view. Our concluding goal is more modest. Each chapter's discussion illuminates a vast territory, yet the extent of our present ignorance about the potential for reducing the cost of dental care remains great. Every chapter, explicitly or implicitly, suggests further research that could significantly narrow the realm of that ignorance. Thus, after presenting a brief summary of each of the chapters, we will identify critical research topics related directly to the subject of the chapter.

MARKET FORCES

How do supply, demand, and the market structure within which dental services are delivered interact with one another to determine dental costs? How will changes in these factors significantly affect dental-care costs during the next decade? Conrad and Milgrom face the ambitious task of answering these questions first by addressing aspects of the supply of dental services. They disagreed with econometric modeling by the Health Resources Administration, which had forecast a gradual substitution of dentists' time for that of auxiliaries' over the period 1978-1995. The HRA position was based on the assumption that increased competition in the dental marketplace would cause a reduction in the implicit relative price of the dentist's own time and that this would be intensified by further competitive pressure from dental advertising and nontraditional practitioners, such as denturists and independent dental hygienists. Believing that the HRA forecasts have overstated the shift away from auxiliary employment, the authors postulate that dental schools are likely to reduce their enrollments in response to declines in the federal subsidies for dental students and that the rate of return to training will not remain high enough to ensure that the number of dental graduates will be determined by dental-school capacity. Citing examples from research studies, the authors conclude that auxiliary-intensive practice will continue to be a reasonable strategy for cost reduction.

The Federal Trade Commission, with an eye toward increased access as well as price competition, supported, until recently, the concept of independent practice of dental hygiene. Conrad and Milgrom believe that this could become a significant way to reduce the unit costs of providing prophylaxis, oral hygiene instruction, and perhaps sealants. But the quantitative impact on the entire system is questionable; a 1977 study indicated that these procedures reflected less than 7 percent of the dentist's total income. It is more likely that greater economies will be realized through the evolution of group and large-scale practices. One of the barriers to achieving technical efficiency in large-scale practices arises from the lack of individual incentives to produce. In addition, the nature of those who select dentistry as a career and their ability to manage large-scale practices complicates the issue.

Nondentist ownership of dental practices may be a feasible means of providing expertise in the managerial aspects of the delivery system. A partnership between dentistry and industry may provide the means to attain price reductions without sacrificing quality of service. Conrad and Milgrom point out that, although ownership of dental practices by other than licensed dentists is prohibited by most state dental acts, the development of corporate franchising in conjunction with cooperating dentists has resulted in fifty or more dental delivery systems based on "retail outlets." Using advertising as well as auxiliary-intensive and large-scale practices, this form of dental delivery suggests opportunities for improved technical and allocative efficiency.

Although the authors present convincing evidence that current state restrictions on the number of dental offices that a dentist may own (one office in California, two offices in Texas, Iowa, Kentucky, and Connecticut) can be expected to hinder the development of multi-dentist practice networks, the small number of states restricting this activity would not make a significant contribution to cost reduction were the legislation to be relaxed. A similar argument can be made for state practice acts that limit the number of hygienists per dentist. Twelve states limit the number of hygienists, and although results show a small increase in dental-service prices, the hygienists deliver a relatively small proportion of the services. Therefore, it is highly unlikely that repeal of these restrictions would have significant impact on price.

Since dentists operate in an environment that allows almost total diagnostic freedom (e.g., free of secondary opinions except when submitting claims for third-party payment), it has been hypothesized that they have the ability to partially control their incomes by raising total dental expenditures. The authors contest this hypothesis with data that appear inconsistent with the target-income hypothesis. Rather, they suggest that increases in the supply of dental practitioners are likely to have a moderating effect on the full price of dental services.

Conrad and Milgrom also address a subject of common concern throughout the United States. The increasing real cost of energy will increase the importance of convenient locations for people to purchase their dental care. Practices that now draw from a wide geographic area can be expected to lose patients to those practices with a more concentrated patient population. This may eventually result in a downward adjustment of the fees of dentists in disadvantageous locations. In addition, it is predicted that multiple appointments for dental procedures will be reduced and that centralization of specialty practices approximating the greatest concentration of generalists will occur in order to minimize travel costs.

Turning to demand factors, the authors point out that the *Bates* decision 1974 and its subsequent effects have already affected dentistry. The American Dental Association, under attack by the FTC for hindering competition, changed position by mid-1979 to allow for truthful advertising by dentists. The authors suggest that advertising will have a major impact on dental-care costs through: (1)

increased competition among providers; (2) growth of franchised and retail-based dental practices and large-scale dental firms; and (3) changes in the mix of dental services as advertising-induced competition alters relative prices.

Increased market competition would encourage greater technical efficiency within the existing practice configurations. Thus, advertising is likely to speed the evolution of the market toward larger, lower-cost dental firms. This should introduce into the dental marketplace individuals who had previously been nonusers, thus increasing total demand. This increase should raise dental expenditure levels even after accounting for a drop in price for present services. The authors hypothesize that persuasive advertising by individual dental practices is less likely to be used effectively for primary dental-care services, which are purchased repetitively as part of an ongoing provider-patient relationship, than for one-time specialty services such as orthodontics. The authors suggest that institutional advertising by the American Dental Association will ultimately strengthen the competitiveness of the entire dental-care sector.

The final portion of the Conrad and Milgrom chapter concerns the growth of prepaid dental plans in the United States. The phenomenal growth of prepaid dental insurance from five million participants in 1972 to seventy million a decade later means that there has been little time to study this issue carefully. However, certain features of prepaid dental insurance seem apparent:

1. On average, per capita expenditures will at least double under full coverage, based on the impact of dental coverage on frequency of visits alone; allowing for adjustments to service mix is likely to increase the estimated expenditure effect.
2. By reducing the proportion of costs borne by patients at the point of service, dental coverage greatly reduces the price sensitivity of demand. Thus, dental-care coverage will shift consumer concerns in the direction of comparative provider amenities, quality, and convenience of time and travel. On the supply side these insurance effects will induce a shift of competitive effort from price margins to the nonprice dimensions of dental care.
3. The burden of cost containment in the dental-care sector thus falls increasingly on the prepayment plan.

Conrad and Milgrom continue their discussion by addressing the overall question of cost reduction and market forces. They point out that risk reduction has less value for prepaid dental plans than for hospital and medical insurance. Meaningful cost control by prepaid dental plans must address the control of claim costs. Present methods include the use of deductibles, coinsurance, pretreatment review, and, until recently, radiographic evidence for posttreatment review. A related factor is the impact of the federal exemption for health—including dental—insurance.

Conrad and Milgrom conclude that "to remove collective restraints on market alternatives, whether in the form of ethical codes or legal statutes, is consistent with a subtle society-wide shift in favor of private incentives as opposed to command-and-control mechanisms for allocating resources."

Critical Research Areas

1. The impact of increasing numbers of female dentists on dental labor markets.
2. The impact of the removal of employer-paid dental health insurance tax exemption on competition and dental-care costs.
3. The cost-containing capacity of HMOs.
4. Advertising's impact on the dental marketplace.
5. The growth of franchise dental practices, particularly, whom they serve and at what cost.
6. The cost-reducing potential of the independent practice of dental hygiene.

THE DELIVERY OF DENTAL CARE

This chapter is based on some key specifications and assumptions: there is no one delivery system for dental care in the United States; rather there are many different subsystems, oftentimes in competition with one another. Bailit and Kudrle further assume that at the aggregate level, provision of more dental services leads to more dental health.

The first substantive section of the paper deals with provider incentives and the cost of care. Although solo practice continues to dominate, an increasing amount of United States dentistry is delivered either in partnerships or in group practices. Very few of the latter include more than five dentists. Practices where one dentist employs others are becoming more common in urban centers, particularly where the owner employs extensive advertising. Most of dentistry continues to be provided on a fee-for-service basis; in fact less than 1 percent of all practices are involved in capitation plans.

Approximately five million people are eligible for treatment in the

Process-level regulations are frequently employed by both private and public bodies. The most familiar are used by insurance companies to avoid the overutilization of expensive services. Sometimes specific services are excluded; other frequently employed devices are the requirement that all treatment above a certain dollar figure be preauthorized on the basis of radiographs and the use of fee screens. The direct and indirect effects of insurance monitoring are estimated to save perhaps 20 percent on overall treatment costs. It is possible that these procedures may improve the efficiency of the production of dental health in some cases by pointing dentists toward more cost-effective procedures. The greater use of practice profiles in system monitoring could increase this effect.

The trend toward locating dental practices where people spend their workdays is a potentially important development. More convenient sites might result in fewer broken or missed appointments and thus increased efficiency; convenient siting is certainly critical to new treatment modalities that involve many brief treatments over the year. Convenient treatment cannot be counted on to reduce total dental-care expenditures; indeed such expenditures would probably increase.

Expansion of school-based dental clinics for poor people has been limited by lack of funds and the opposition of the dental profession. Medicaid offers a potential answer to the problem for those schools in which many of the students are eligible. Where facilities already exist, private dentists could deliver such services in the schools.

An alternative to the present system or the one just proposed would be for private dental firms to contract with school boards to provide care in schools with large, eligible populations. The firms could have five-year contracts and would provide their own capital equipment. Maximum contact could be established and maximum incentive for all preventive services could be engendered if the firm were paid on a capitation basis. A variant on this system would be for the public authority to provide the capital equipment.

A final school-based innovation would involve minimum change in the present private-practice-based Medicaid system. Only inspection would take place in the school; subsequently, the student's own dentist would notify the family of the condition and eligibility for public payment. The system could be expanded to include all of the children to a certain age, regardless of eligibility for public benefits. Such school inspections are, of course, dental-health and not cost-containment measures unless combined with preventive interventions.

Cost reduction also includes the possibility of patient strategies.

Individuals as patients can seek out the lowest cost sources of dental treatment for any given level of quality. Individuals as citizens can work for public policies directed toward providing better quality or lower-cost dental care. Some legislative changes proposed in the early 1980s might reduce the tax incentives for cost-containment problems that now stem from the absence of patient and practitioner attention to costs under dental insurance.

Bailit and Kudrle conclude that very large increases in efficiency do not appear likely solely from reorganization of the dental-care delivery system under present legal conditions. This conclusion must be distinguished from the impact on the price of services resulting from the greater availability of dental manpower and increased competition. Dramatic cost breakthroughs may await advancement in the science of treatment. There are, however, a few other cost-reducing possibilities. The greater use of Expanded Function Dental Auxiliaries (EFDAs) to do both reversible and irreversible procedures, might greatly lower costs of treatment if EFDAs were legal and the competitive environment obliged dentistry to employ them. Third-party payers might attempt to lower their expenditures on dental care by limiting the payment allowed for procedures; this practice could only exist, of course, where dentists depend on these payers for a large part of their income.

Future technical breakthroughs may require changes in the delivery system. The development of an anti-plaque agent that must be applied quarterly could well have this impact. Finally, it is likely that both lowered production costs and prices and more effective treatment will increase, rather than reduce, total dental-care expenditures.

Critical Research Areas

1. The patterns of treatment in capitation plans and their impact on costs and dental health compared to fee-for-service.
2. The extent to which insurance benefits can significantly affect dental health.
3. The efficacy and delivery-system implications of frequent preventive interventions using representative American adults.
4. The viability of leasing dental facilities in schools to private dental firms.
5. The effectiveness of using school inspections in a dental benefit plan followed by private office treatment.

AUXILIARY PERSONNEL

Born's historical approach describes the use of auxiliary personnel in dentistry in a development context. Among the input factors affecting cost in the delivery of services, labor is the most critical. Assuming that qulaity is maintained, Born considers several labor inputs that might be substituted for those of the dentist but at a lower cost.

Historically, dentists have found and used less expensive labor resources for certain tasks associated with patient care and practice administration. Over 100 years of experience have clearly demonstrated the efficacy of using auxiliaries. The advantages generally include stress reduction, lower production costs, and increased output. Yet, in retrospect, changes that might reasonably be expected in response to such advantages have come only slowly. For example, ten to fifteen years passed before a majority of dentists were persuaded to practice "sit-down, four-handed" dentistry rather than the "stand-up, solo" style that was popular into the sixties.

Although from a managerial perspective dentistry has evolved slowly, Born notes that following World War II, many socioeconomic forces influenced dental leaders, educators, and government policymakers. Among these were an increased interest in the benefits of technology; an almost evangelistic faith in the power of systematic, quantitative management science as a solution to social as well as industrial problems; increased funding of programs designend to eliminate inate social and health-care delivery problems; expectations of increased health-care demand; and forecasts of an impending health-care crisis.

Responding to these influences, the profession, the dental schools, and the government united in a variety of innovative ventures designed to increase the capacity of the dental sector. Two key developments resulted from those activities. First, both dental and auxiliary program graduates were increased sharply within a single decade. Second, extensive documentation was compiled on the productivity advances that are possible using traditional and experimental personnel mixes in a variety of dental-care delivery settings.

A third, more subtle outcome also evolved: auxiliary personnel themselves became more fully aware of the impact they could have as employees and as "independent" dental-care providers. Thus, an expanded auxiliary workforce with heightened expectations was created simultaneously with the expansion of the dentist workforce. If the expected "boom" in dental-care demand had materialized, these socioeconomic forces might have evened themselves out; but with the economic downturn of the mid-seventies, the profession found itself on the brink of a supply "overload"—a productive capacity in excess of demand.

Born also suggests that dentists comprise a rigidly socialized profession that has been able to maintain monopolistic control over the dental industry. Since dentistry is practiced through a great many independent firms, output cannot be controlled directly. Instead, the socialization process and the close-knit nature of the profession enable it to exercise great control over the training, licensing, and employment of both dentists and auxiliaries. In this way, supply is controlled. Born argues that dentists protect each other (consciously or unconsciously) by managing relatively small, moderately efficient practices — practices that will give them a modest share of the market without cutting the (economic) throats of their colleagues.

This historical background and Born's comments on dentistry's self-protective market control are important to his views on the issue of cost containment and auxiliary utilization. They provide the perspective from which Born focuses his attention on four categories of auxiliaries: denturists, EFDAs, independently practicing dental hygienists, and indirectly supervised EFDAs such as "school dental nurses."

Rising from the ranks of dental laboratory technicians, denturists have rallied hard in recent years for recognition as health-care providers in their own right. As the manufacturers of dentures and other prosthetic dental devices, denturists have argued that they are technically capable of dealing directly with the public and that in such transactions, consumers can realize substantial savings (by eliminating the dentist as middleman).

According to Born, the major threat to dentists is that denturists will succeed in obtaining legal recognition as *independent* providers of denture services (as they have indeed done in Oregon). Under these circumstances, denturists would be freed from the constraints that control all other dental-care providers and could conceivably compete aggressively with dentists for a portion of the denture market. Bleak as that outlook might sound to most dentists, Born's prognosis is that an independent denturist "profession," once established, will follow the example of its "big brother" and attempt to exercise monopolistic controls over its share of the market.

Born contends, then, that significant cost containment is not likely to result from the licensing of denturists unless they can be kept independent of dentists and unless they can be prevented from developing monopolistic controls such as those found in dentistry.

The author proceeds with the wealth of evidence supporting EFDAs as highly effective labor substitutes that, if utilized appropriately, could help achieve major cost reduction. Such savings are not likely at present, says Born, again citing the particular characteristics of the dental profession. Individual dentists can practice only in a moderately efficient manner because to do otherwise might further unleash rampant competition. Should such competition emerge, the entire nature of dental practice would be altered and many professionals could end up being forced out of business by highly efficient operators expanding into the market.

Independent dental hygienists and indirectly supervised EFDAs (along the lines of school dental nurses) are considered offshoots from the same series of developments that led to emergence of four-handed dentistry and expanded functions for auxiliaries. Although other factors are involved, neither group possesses significant political power when faced with the dental profession's rigid control. Why should the profession, faced with excess capacity in a lagging economy, relinquish its monopolistic control by supporting the development of independent (or quasi-independent) dental care providers?

In conclusion, Born suggests that, while significant advances in the area of cost containment are possible via auxiliary utilization, widespread use of auxiliaries will become likely only as external economic forces trigger major competitive struggles. Otherwise, divisive competitive forces would drastically threaten dentistry as today's dentists know it.

Born suggests that major structural pressures within the dental marketplace, such as the purported surplus of dentists or innovative delivery systems spawned by third-party agencies, might trigger the changes that the author feels are necessary if cost reductions are to be realized through efficient use of auxiliary personnel.

Critical Research Areas

1. The impact on price and quality of denturism in Canada.
2. Optimal auxiliary staffing patterns for different case mixes and patient loads.
3. An impact study on competition and cost if the independent practice of dental hygiene becomes legal.
4. Management systems appropriate for maximizing the use of expanded function auxiliaries.

COST CONTAINMENT IN DENTAL EDUCATION

Rovin, Scheffler, and Bauer claim that dentistry is facing a crisis in the education of its professionals, a crisis shared by other health professionals. The authors identify two major areas that they believe offer the potential of cost reduction in dental education. The first is the cost of providing dental education itself; the second issue is the long-term effect of the type of dental education on the cost of dental care. While the immediate and long-term concerns about cost may appear independent, numerous examples in the chapter indicate that concurrent changes can be complementary.

As federal support declines, a continued rise in indebtedness may force dentists to seek higher gross incomes by increasing fees, providing more expensive services, increasing the number of their services, and working longer hours. However, it is also possible that because of high educational debt and high initial practice costs students may seek salaried or other nonentrepreneurial practice modes.

Because of the increasing expense of becoming a dentist, applications to dental school have declined, a trend that is expected to continue. Using the concept of the economic rate-of-return to training, the authors demonstrate that there is a direct relationship between the rate-of-return to training (RRT) and the number of applications over the years 1960-1970 and in 1977. Since the chapter addresses solutions as well as problems, the RRT concept is used to test the impact of shortening or lengthening dental training. This concept may be useful in future dental-education planning.

Rovin, Scheffler, and Bauer also comment on the potential change in the composition of applications to dental school. Although a decline in quality of students as the result of fewer applications has not yet been a concern, it is conceivable that minority groups, who have finally seen barriers to their entry into dental school lowered, may now find that the high cost of education and the potential debt, as well as the lowered RRT, do not make dentistry an attractive profession. Since many of these individuals have come from ethnic and racial groups that have had to depend on the nonminority dentist for services, these groups would have to continue this pattern.

The authors offer six means by which to cope with increasing indebtedness and enrollment problems. Arguing that dentists who graduate at forty or forty-five years of age are as capable as those who graduate at twenty-five, the authors contend that these individuals might have the financial wherewithal to pay for a dental education without incurring the debt assumed by the younger applicant. Self-paced curricula allowing students to attend on a work-study basis for longer periods of time is another approach; it includes the concept of night-school classes that might permit minority students to continue their quest for a professional education. A third solution is the reinstatement of early graduation for students who demonstrate suitable competency. A shortened educational period would have an obvious effect on the RRT. To increase the number of applicants, the authors suggest that dental schools might engage in advertising the benefits of dental education. They also suggest that a consolidation of present dental schools, through closing or merging, would create a more cost-effective dental education system. A complementary strategy is regionalization, in which schools would divide certain specialty programs to achieve cost-effective education. The sixth suggestion is the introduction of innovative, alternative fiscal mechanisms to amortize student loans, either over a long period of time, or to provide tax incentives or tuition forgiveness.

The issue of the supply of dentists and the effect that supply may have on price is integral to this discussion. The authors suggest that it may not be reasonable to act too precipitously to reduce supply, because rises in demand might be generated by increases in third-party payment. Payments by third parties have grown from the coverage of five million people in 1972 to approximately seventy million in 1981; in addition, 50 percent of the population still does not see a dentist on a yearly basis. Rovin, Scheffler, and Bauer argue that a reduction in production of manpower would make no contribution to cost reduction and could contribute to cost escalation. The authors contend that the best option is to change the mix of dental manpower through a decrease in specialty training, an expansion of the scope of the general dentist, and a greater emphasis on auxiliary training. This system would be flexible enough to meet any short-term increases in demand and at the same time would reduce overall expenditures on dental education by reducing costs of training. In this regard, the authors join Conrad and Milgrom in questioning a recent HEW publication that predicts a decline in the employment of auxiliaries because of an increase in practice time among dentists. An auxiliary-intensive practice would be more profitable and cost effective, the authors believe. It is their general view that a flexible delivery system coupled with an emphasis on health care rather than disease care (the former desired, but the latter prevailing) would reorient the entire educational process and introduce new reward systems for preventing rather than treating disease. More curriculum time in acquiring the skills for and inculcating attitudes toward prevention is needed, as is a reorientation of faculty attitudes and skills. Although the authors are doubtful that the profession is easily capable of making such changes, they do believe that to survive in the future, dental education must emphasize health care more than disease care.

The organization and management of dental schools are critical both to the cost of supplying education and to the attitudes that dental practitioners carry from the schools. The authors argue that innovative cooperation and change must be a precondition for survival of dental education. If schools use the philosophy that form follows function, an alteration in their function will make it easier to alter organizational structures. They contend that success will require the subordination of departmental interests to school-wide interests in the coming years.

Along with these organizational changes, Rovin, Scheffler, and Bauer argue that people who manage dental-school, patient-care enterprises are often ill-equipped for the managerial aspects of their jobs. Perhaps a nondentist or a dentist working in conjunction with a management-trained person could promote progress and harmony in this vital area. Another crucial consideration is the faculty, a group which the authors believe is not being used efficiently. They propose a clinical educator track for full-time faculty and more efficient use of part-time faculty. They hope to accomplish the latter by employing an incentive plan that would reimburse part-time teachers on the basis of the performance of the students under their direction. Finally, an examination of the tenure code would be conducted and, if necessary, redefined.

Patient care in dental-school facilities is described as inefficient and cost-ineffective. With increases in third-party payment and the number of available dentists, many dental schools are suffering precipitous drops in available patients in certain clinical areas of instruction. According to the authors, the present system serves providers (students and faculty) and not consumers.

Dental schools must adopt the philosophy that patient care is their primary goal. Education by necessity must become a byproduct. The ultimate responsibility for patient care would reside with faculty members and not with the students, state the authors, adding that a faculty member's income would be at least partially dependent on this provision of care. Furthering their argument, the authors believe that students could become part of this system and share in the income generated, thus reducing their cost of education. For this kind of system to evolve, dental schools might have to decentralize and actually become partners with existing dental offices where students and practitioners would work side-by-side. Furthermore, the authors contend, the dental curriculum must change along with the structure. Students, who are now taught to perform the highest quality of dental care regardless of cost, must learn to perform the highest quality of dentistry commensurate with a reasonable cost so that the system may compete in the present marketplace.

In conclusion, Rovin, Scheffler, and Bauer emphasize that the eighties are crucial for reform and innovation. Maintaining the status quo in the dental profession will provide neither education nor patient care at reasonable cost.

Critical Research Areas

1. The impact of the cost of education and expected income on numbers and types of student applications. One approach to the first issue would be to compare high-tuition private schools with public schools.
2. The cost and division-of-labor possibilities of the regionalization of dental education.
3. Possibilities for the introduction of cost-sensitive curricula in dental schools.
4. The feasibility of faculty incentive systems (faculty-owned practices and faculty- and university-owned practices).
5. Innovative ways to finance educational costs for dental students.
6. The potential of sharing clinic income with faculty and students.

PREVENTION

Burt and Warner's chapter introduction quickly establishes one fundamental truth: increasing prevention does not necessarily translate into increasing future cost-savings. From that starting-point, the authors present their working definition of cost containment as the most reasonable minimization of all costs associated with dental care, including those costs associated with a failure to receive needed dental care. Their concept comprises not only minimization of direct expenditures on dental care, but, more unusually, takes account of such costs as time required for treatment; they also include the personal and social costs of dental neglect and other aspects of the loss of quality of life brought about by dental disease.

The authors suggest that prevention of dental disease presents a conceptually attractive approach to reducing costs. The basis for this appeal is simple: relatively low-cost investments in disease prevention will prevent or postpone the onset of disease that may lead to tooth loss or expensive care. The dental disease are dental caries and periodontal disease. Knowledge and procedures are available to individuals and professionals for the prevention of both diseases.

Examination of the cost-reduction potential of prevention must include a consideration of outcomes, although there are limitations imposed by the lack of knowledge of lifelong effectiveness of most preventive procedures. From the available evidence, Burt and Warner conclude that procedures with most promise for life-long retention of teeth are water fluoridation and regular periodic professional plaque removal combined with patient education.

To illustrate the impact of prevention, Burt and Warner develop seven cost streams of necessarily simplified lifetime dental histories, a cost stream being a sequence of annual expenditures for dental care over the lifetime of a hypothetical individual. Each cost stream assumes various combinations of preventive procedures, treatment histories, and dental-health outcomes. The seven cost streams are:

A. Total neglect, loss of all teeth by age thirty-five to thirty-nine.
B. Water fluoridation, regular annual care in youth, less regular care in adulthood without special periodontal emphasis. Loss of all teeth by age seventy to seventy-four.
C. No water fluoridation, regular annual care in youth, less regular care in adulthood without special periodontal emphasis. Loss of all teeth by age fifty-five to fifty-nine.
D. Water fluoridation, regular annual care in youth, quarterly care in adulthood with periodontal emphasis in the form of quarterly professional cleanings (as defined by Lindhe and Axelsson in 1974) provided by a dentist or highly trained auxiliary. Loss of one tooth by age thirty-five, no more thereafter.
E. No water fluoridation, regular annual care in youth, quarterly care in adulthood with periodontal emphasis in the form of quarterly professional cleanings provided by a dentist or highly trained auxiliary. Loss of three teeth by age thirty-five, no more thereafter.
F. Water fluoridation, regular annual care in youth, quarterly care in adulthood with periodontal emphasis in the form of quarterly professional cleanings provided by a lesser-trained auxiliary. Loss of one tooth by age thirty-five, no more thereafter (assuming that the quality of care provided by the auxiliary is similar to that of the dentist).
G. No water fluoridation, regular annual care in youth, quarterly care in adulthood with periodontal emphasis in the form of quarterly professional cleanings provided by a lesser-trained auxiliary (again assuming that the quality of the care provided by the auxiliary is similar to that of the dentist). Loss of three teeth by age thirty-five, no more thereafter.

Dental treatment provided is expressed in the form of Relative Value Units (RVUs) for ease of quantification. These RVUs are then converted to 1977 dollar values for care received. These dollar values are then discounted to allow expression of lifetime expenditures in terms of their present value. The lifetime expenditures in each of the seven streams are then comparable.

The authors made no attempt to quantify those areas mentioned in the broader definition of cost containment stated at the beginning, that is, the indirect costs related to quality of life. Although some quality-of-life impacts are implicit in the variable outcomes of the seven cost streams, Burt and Warner admit the difficulty of attempting to establish dollar values for effects in areas such as personal and social quality of life.

The authors' results show that the lowest direct expenditures for lifetime dental treatment are required in cost stream A, total neglect. If the narrow view of cost minimization is taken, it follows that complete neglect would be the course to follow. Such a recommendation is socially and culturally unacceptable, and may in addition be poor economics because the costs of pain, poor appearance, and other intangibles have not been considered. But to dismiss this finding solely on cost grounds, it is necessary to adopt the broader definition of cost containment stated at the outset.

The broad view of cost minimization also needs to be borne in mind when considering the other results. The next least-expensive care noted was in cost stream B, fluoridation and total tooth loss at age seventy to seventy-four, followed by cost stream F, fluoridation and no loss of teeth in adulthood. Although cost stream B requires less direct expenditure, there is the intangible cost of total tooth loss. Cost stream F also demands a more elaborate pattern of dental visits throughout life, itself a cost. Burt and Warner conclude that total prevention of disease over a lifetime is probably impossible for most people. What is possible for many of these same people, they claim, is substantial prevention of caries and control of periodontal disease to a point where inflammation is minor and loss of bony support minimized. If this relatively limited goal can be accepted, then the nature of lifetime prevention in a cost-reduction context becomes clearer.

Critical Research Areas

1. Economic and social incentives for prevention, including lower insurance rates in fluoridated areas.
2. Research into short- and long-term outcomes as a result of different preventive interventions.

3. Impact of institutional and professional advertising on the acceptance and utilization of preventive procedures.
4. Further extension of the Burt-Warner model to include travel and treatment time and social considerations.
5. Selective application of preventive procedures to high-risk school populations.

QUALITY ASSURANCE

Quality of care is assumed to be an important characteristic of dental care, but, as is the case in medicine, it has proved difficult to define satisfactorily. Quality can be considered in structure, process, and outcome dimensions, each of which presents formidable definitional and measurement problems. Quality assessment is the term usually used for measuring the quality of care provided, while the term quality assurance is used to refer to stepwise processes used to rectify identified deficiencies.

In the policy realm, Marcus and Tobin break down the problems of quality assurance into four categories: the technical quality of care, the art of care, overutilization, and underutilization. Interestingly, the relation between poor technical quality of care and dental health is poorly understood. In some areas the connection is clear and dramatic—in others there appears to be rather little connection.

The considerations that must be factored into any decision to introduce a quality-assurance system include: the extent to which unacceptable care is prevalent, the effects of unacceptable care on the dental health of the population, the costs of implementing a quality-assurance system, and its ability to resolve the problem of technical quality.

Quality-assurance activities combine steps that involve the review of claims, patients, or practices. In presently functioning systems, often operated by third-party payers, it is difficult to separate program administrative functions—the designation of benefits—from quality-assurance activities. Although quality-assurance systems may be operated by either public or private organizations and can assume either a professional or a directly financial orientation, the main activity so far has been at the initiative of private financial organizations. Nonetheless, the American Dental Association (and its constituent societies) has taken some steps to survey the state of the quality of dental care in the United States and has established its own review committees to work in conjunction with prepayment schemes. The American Fund for Dental Health and the Kellogg Foundation have established a National Dental Quality Assurance Advisory Committee to study "a national program of quality assurance in Dentistry." Public professional quality-assurance activities include the licensure of professionals and health-care plans, quality control in public programs, and publicly funded research activities that bear on quality and quality control.

In analyzing the market forces that produce the observed levels of service and quality, it must be remembered that three distinct parties with different interests are involved: patients, dentists, and third-party payers. There is presently insufficient information on the extent to which the incentives under which providers operate lead them to provide sufficient information to the patient about the cost-quality tradeoff. One role of quality assurance, of course, is to help the consumer be better prepared to select a certain point on the cost-quality frontier, and to ensure that the quality selected is actually delivered. Formally, one would like to see quality assurance provided to the point that the marginal benefit of such assurance just matches its marginal cost.

It is almost certain that the increasing level of third-party payment in dentistry has increased both the volume of services delivered and the quality of those services. The provision of insurance typically creates a quality as well as quantity distortion among both patients and dentists. Not only do insured patients consume more dental services than they would otherwise, but dentists and patients have an incentive to increase the quality as well. Nonetheless, if the provision of an insurance plan provides for meager reimbursement to providers, the quality of insured dental care may suffer.

The chapter's Appendix discusses models of quality assurance based on differing assumptions about the public-insurance scheme under which the assurance system would operate. Although the numbers are illustrative only, they are based on actual data compiled for an elaborate government-sponsored study. The model operates on a set of equations that contains requests made in the program, a linking generator, and the quality-assurance system itself. The model handles nine major service categories. The system assumes either a high-benefit plan in which 39.9 percent of all services are crown and bridge work or a low-benefit plan in which only 2.0 percent are crown and bridge.

The Appendix to Chapter 6 also develops a model in which policy-makers can simultaneously model the efficacy of the quality-assurance system, the technical quality of the services produced in the system being monitored (a consideration ignored in the previous exercise), and the extent of over-, under-, or appropriate utilization. A combination of best estimates of these variables and a policymaker's own evaluation of how much various corrective measure are worth can help illuminate the central issue of whether a quality-assurance system is really worth introducing in a public program. These evaluative weights can and should include both financial and health-related costs and benefits.

For illustrative purposes the text discusses in detail the operation of quality assurance for claims authorization. The claims-review process has two dimensions: one involving administrative judgment is simply whether the service requested is in fact covered. This judgment has no implications for quality assurance, but the ones involving professional judgment do. The latter result from practitioner requests for preauthorization for certain procedures. The practitioner may propose one kind of treatment, but the consulting professional may suggest another on either economic or dental-health grounds. If the practitioner disputes the determinations of the consultant, the decision can be appealed, in which case a consultant gives the patient a direct examination. If the matter is still not settled to the practitioner's satisfaction, the matter can be appealed further. The process ends with a peer review committee (representing the profession) and an arbitration board whose decision is final.

What would one hope for from this system concerning quality rather than cost? If the monitoring system's judgments are correct, the dental health of the patient whose case is being directly dealt with is enhanced, while at the same time, an educational function is being performed for the practitioner. But if the system is wrong, the patient-dentist relationship has been complicated, not for a greater good, but with an additional negative effect on the final outcome. Overall, the significance of the quality-assurance system is seen in the model to vary depending on the nature of the requests, the extent of problems encountered, and the vigilance of the system itself.

Critical Research Areas

1. The extent of technically inferior treatment being delivered in American dentistry.
2. The relation of the art-of-care to personal disease-prevention behavior.
3. The extent to which patients can and do understand the nature of cost-quality tradeoffs in dentistry.
4. The extent of over- and undertreatment in American dentistry.
5. The effectiveness of various kinds of quality-assurance systems

in actually providing defensible treatment judgment, and the associated costs of each system.

A CONCLUDING NOTE ON GOVERNMENT POLICY

No one knows what the future holds for dentistry. Fifteen or fewer years ago, positive action by the federal government in supporting dental education and introducing dental benefits into public programs was profoundly affecting dentistry and appeared to be the biggest unknown in dentistry's future. Federal government action remains almost certainly the greatest wild card in the entire system. The government's determination to expand dental-practitioner supply has contributed strongly to a large supply relative to demand and quite possibly a long period of unprecedentedly low incomes for dental practitioners. Furthermore, it is as yet unclear whether the withdrawal of the federal government from most of its positive activity to increase dentist supply will result in a major decrease in the output of dental schools or simply in lower income expectations among dentists—and perhaps a change in the profile of persons going into dentistry.

This vast expansion of dentist supply was, perhaps unwittingly, a strongly "pro-competitive" act by the federal government. Moreover, recent actions by the FTC are part of a society-wide rejection of professional autonomy. The growing tide of advertising will certainly not be turned back, and independent practice by nondentists will continue to receive careful attention. Finally—and this was scarcely predicted until very recently—the growth of third-party payment might be halted or reversed by a removal of the opportunity for employees to receive untaxed income in the form of dental insurance. This, in turn, could have a major effect on both the total demand for dental services and the extent of price competition in dental-care markets.

Few observers—including those writing this book—believe that government-spending initiatives for dental care are likely in the eighties. Yet the pivotal role of the government remains. Implicitly or explicitly, most of the authors in this book suggest that the degree of price reduction and production-cost-saving innovation will be directly related to the extent of competition experienced in dentistry. And the definition and enforcement of this competition will remain in the hands of state and federal agencies.

Index

Index

215

Robert T. Kudrle, an associate professor in the
Hubert H. Humphrey Institute of Public Affairs
at the University of Minnesota, is an economist, one
of whose specialties is health care policy. He is co-
editor of *International Studies Quarterly* and a
member of the editorial board of the *Journal of
Health Politics, Policy and Law.* **Lawrence Meskin,**
D.D.S., was chairman of the department of health
ecology in the dental school at the University of
Minnesota from 1970 to 1981 and is now dean of
the dental school at the University of Colorado. Long
committed to the public-health and preventive
aspects of dental care, he has served as a consultant
to the Division of Dental Health, United States
Public Health Service, and to the Pan American and
World Health Organizations in the Caribbean basin.